Janet
1994.

M000159768

Cumulative trauma disorders:
A manual for musculoskeletal diseases
of the upper limbs

Cumulative trauma disorders: A manual for musculoskeletal diseases of the upper limbs

Edited by
Vern Putz-Anderson

National Institute for Occupational Safety and Health,
Cincinnati, Ohio, USA

Taylor & Francis

USA   Taylor & Francis Inc., 1900 Frost Road, Suite 101, Bristol, PA 19007

UK   Taylor & Francis Ltd, 4 John St., London WC1N 2ET

Copyright © Taylor & Francis Ltd 1988

Reprinted 1990, 1991, 1992

All rights reserved. No part of this publication may be reproduced, stored in a retrieval system, or transmitted, in any form or by any means, electronic, mechanical, photocopying, recording or otherwise, without the prior permission of the copyright owner and publishers.

British Library Cataloguing in Publication Data

Cumulative trauma disorders: a manual for musculoskeletal diseases of the upper limbs.
  1. Vibration—Physiological effect.   2. Hand—Wounds and injuries.
  3. Arm—Wounds and injuries.   4. Industrial injuries.
  I. Putz-Anderson, Vern
  617'.57   RC963.5.V5

  ISBN 0-85066-405-5

Library of Congress Cataloging in Publication Data

Cumulative trauma disorders: manual for musculoskeletal diseases of the upper limbs/editor, Vern Putz-Anderson,

    p.   cm.
  Bibliography: p.
  Includes index.
  ISBN 0-85066-405-5 (pbk.)
    1. Extremities, upper—Wounds and injuries—Handbooks, manuals, Work injuries, etc. 2. Extremities, Upper—Wounds and injuries—Prevention—Handbooks, manuals, etc. 3. Occupaitonal diseases—Prevention—Handbooks, manuals, etc. 4. Disability evaluation—Handbooks, manuals, etc. I. Putz-Anderson, Vern.
    [DNLM: 1. Accidents, Occupational—prevention & control. 2. Arm Injuries—diagnosis. 3. Arm Injuries—prevention & control. 4. Disability Evaluation.
WE 805 C971]
RD557.C86   1988
617'.57044—dc19
DNLM/DLC   87-33569
for Library of Congress   CIP

Cover design by Ray Eves
Illustration by Al Tudor

Typeset by Alresford Typesetting & Design, New Farm Road, Alresford, Hants.

Printed in Great Britain by Burgess Science Press, Rankine Road, Basingstoke, Hants.

Reprinted in the United States by Braun-Brumfield, Inc.

Contents

Abstract

This manual was developed to define cumulative trauma disorders (CTDs) in the workplace, to enable non-medical personnel to recognize them, and to present strategies for preventing their occurrence. Emphasis is placed on CTDs of the upper extremities.

Part I of this manual defines the cumulative trauma category of musculoskeletal disorders. Information is provided on the structures of the hand and arm to help identify the symptoms and location of the disorders. Descriptions of some of the common types of CTDs are also provided along with examples of jobs in which CTDs may occur.

Part II presents methods for determining how many workers at a worksite have CTDs or have some early symptoms of CTDs. Extensive information on conducting an ergonomic job analysis is also provided. Information from such a job analysis is useful for identifying work conditions and tools that may cause or contribute to CTDs.

Part III focuses on two strategies used to control or prevent the occurrence of CTDs: *Instituting Personnel-Focused Practices* and *Redesigning Tools, Work Stations and Jobs*. The merits of each strategy are discussed. Combinations of elements of each strategy are frequently used in workplaces where prevention programs for CTDs have been implemented. Guidelines for ergonomic redesign are also provided along with a list of references for further information on ergonomics.

The Appendices include specialized material designed to supplement information contained in the body of the manual. Appendix A includes a glossary of terms and a series of illustrations to define the positions and movements of the body. Appendix B provides an introduction to the diagnostic process used by the medical profession to identify CTDs and a summary of medical procedures used to treat them. Appendix C defines some common epidemiological terms and describes statistical procedures for evaluating the prevalence, incidence, and severity of CTDs. In addition, a series of case histories are provided to illustrate the frequency and costs associated with CTDs among specific work populations.

Preface

This manual evolved out of a project in the Division of Biomedical and Behavioral Science, Applied Psychology and Ergonomics Branch, entitled *Methods For Detecting Cumulative Trauma Injury.*

A literature review indicated that there were several methods for detecting cumulative trauma disorders (CTDs). What was missing was a general reference source or a manual that explained, with a minimum of technical language, the concept of CTDs, the parts of the body affected and the potential causes. Once the reader understands the seriousness and characteristics of CTDs, a description of the most current methods for use in detecting, evaluating and controlling CTDs at the worksite can follow and take on new meaning.

The present manual was prepared with this aim.

The manual consists of three distinctive parts and an appendix. To the extent possible, each of the three parts of the manual is complete with respect to its general purpose. Parts I and II were designed primarily to instruct, whereas Part III and the Appendices were designed as a reference tool for the more advanced users.

Part I provides an overview of CTDs for those individuals unfamiliar with the problem. Part II builds on this introductory base and is directed at those individuals responsible for maintaining the health and productivity of the workforce, as well as those responsible for making preliminary determinations about jobs with a potential for CTDs. The emphasis in Part II is on specifying a set of procedures for identifying and analyzing records and jobs for indicators of cumulative trauma. Part III outlines strategies for controlling CTDs and provides a series of ergonomic-based guidelines for redesigning high risk jobs. Part III should be of particular interest to those practitioners who are responsible for improving and maintaining the safety and health of workers. This may include nurses, physicians, safety engineers, union representatives, industrial hygienists, supervisors, insurance carriers, and even individual workers who are concerned about the problem. Finally, the materials presented in the appendix provide an expanded treatment of a variety of issues related to posture, medical treatment, and surveillance techniques that had been previously presented in a more abbreviated form in the body of the manual.

Most of the information contained in the manual was derived from original source materials provided by noted experts in their fields. A list of the contributors is given on page xi.

Vern Putz-Anderson

Acknowledgements

Appreciation is extended to Mr William Beazley who assisted in preparing the first draft while the project director was on a special assignment. Special appreciation is also extended to Mr Henry Williams who served as a dedicated assistant and provided valuable support in every phase of the preparation of the final two versions of the manual. Dr Alexander Cohen, former Chief of the Applied Psychology and Ergonomics Branch, provided both encouragement and valuable direction in developing the manual content. Finally, the suggestions of Dr Suzanne H. Rodgers, one of the original practitioners in this field, were particularly valuable.

The illustrations were drawn by Mr Al Tudor based on suggestions and guidance provided by the editor, Dr Thomas Armstrong, and William Beazley and Henry Williams. Special appreciation is also extended to Mr Richard Carlson and the staff of the Curriculum Development Branch at NIOSH for preparing the final version of the illustrations for publication.

List of Contributors

Thomas J. Armstrong,
Associate Professor of
Industrial Hygiene,
Department of Environmental
and Industrial Health,
The University of Michigan,
Ann Arbor, Michigan

M.M. Ayoub,
Horn Professor of Industrial
Engineering,
Texas Tech University,
Lubbock, Texas.

Colin G. Drury,
Professor of Industrial
Engineering,
State University of New York at
Buffalo,
Buffalo, New York.

Barbara Silverstein,
Assistant Research Scientist,
School of Public Health,
University of Michigan,
Ann Arbor, Michigan.

Lawrence J. Fine,
Associate Professor of
Occupational Medicine,
School of Public Health,
University of Michigan,
Ann Arbor, Michigan.

William L. Hopkins,
Professor of Psychology,
Department of Human
Development,
The University of Kansas,
Lawrence, Kansas.

W. Monroe Keyserling,
Assistant Professor of
Occupational Safety,
Center for Ergonomics,
The University of Michigan,
Ann Arbor, Michigan.

Vern Putz-Anderson,
Chief, Psychophysiology and
Biomechanics Section,
National Institute for
Occupational
Safety and Health, DHHS,
Cincinnati, Ohio.

Disclaimer

The opinions, findings and conclusions expressed herein are not necessarily those of the National Institute for Occupational Safety and Health, nor does mention of company names or products constitute endorsement by the National Institute for Occupational Safety and Health.

Part I

Recognizing Cumulative Trauma Disorders

The recognition that work may adversely affect health was recorded more than 200 years ago by an Italian physician, Bernardino Ramazinni. He identified two types of workplace hazards: the "harmful character of the materials . . . handled" and "certain violent and irregular motions and unnatural postures of the body, by reason of which the natural structure of the vital machine is so impaired that serious diseases gradually develop therefrom."[1]

The first type of hazard—exposure to hazardous materials—is the best known and persists today despite many recent advances in industrial hygiene and control technology. The second category of hazard, irregular motions and postures, is less well known. Terms such as microtrauma, repeated trauma, or chronic trauma have been used as labels. The adverse health effects that arise from chronic exposure to microtrauma are the subject of this manual, viz., the cumulative trauma disorders (CTDs). Until recently, CTDs commanded comparatively little public attention. Yet there is ample evidence from early medical reports that over the years craftsmen experienced a variety of musculoskeletal disorders associated with their trade. Names such as bricklayer's shoulder, carpenter's elbow, stitcher's wrist, game keeper's thumb, telegraphist's cramp, and cotton-twister's hand represent a sampling of the names used to label such syndromes.[2] A common feature was the element of overuse superimposed on the progressive changes that accompany the normal aging of the body.

One major obstacle that may have contributed to the general lack of awareness and research in these disorders is the lack of reliable occupational-based statistics for documenting the prevalence of these disorders. Estimates that are available have been drawn mainly from data bases that were not designed for surveillance, and consequently provide only limited insight into the epidemiology of the problem. Nevertheless, such reports, combined with findings from individual worksites and industrial clinics, do suggest that the hazard described by Ramazzini as "irregular work motions" accounts for an increasing amount of lost worktime and morbidity.[3]

In response to the growing prevalence of the disorders, there has been renewed research interest in cause and prevention.[4]

Although there are many excellent reports and studies on various aspects of CTDs, few of these are widely read or disseminated. The result is a growing information gap or lack of awareness among many occupational health and safety practitioners, workers, and management as to the nature, extent, and causes of these disorders.

This section of the manual provides an introduction to CTDs designed in part to remedy this deficiency. The nature and scope of CTDs is reviewed. Anatomical structures of the hand and arm that are subject to injury from acute and chronic overuse are described. An overview of the types of CTDs and the patterns of usage that contribute to the disorders are briefly outlined. Finally, a list of jobs is presented where various types of CTDs have been reported.

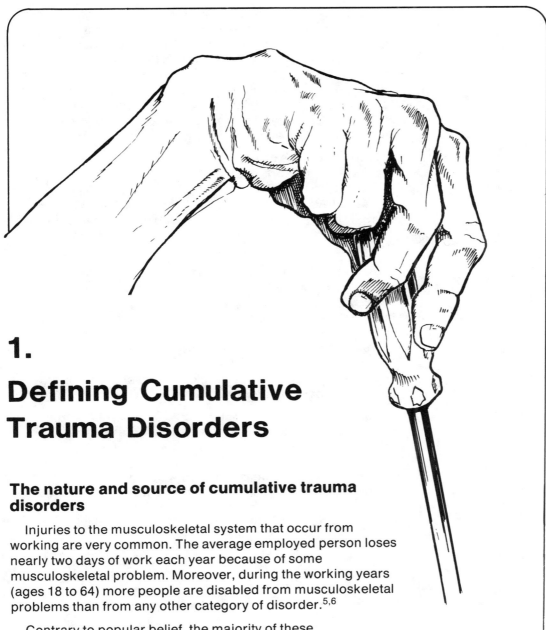

1.

Defining Cumulative Trauma Disorders

The nature and source of cumulative trauma disorders

Injuries to the musculoskeletal system that occur from working are very common. The average employed person loses nearly two days of work each year because of some musculoskeletal problem. Moreover, during the working years (ages 18 to 64) more people are disabled from musculoskeletal problems than from any other category of disorder.[5,6]

Contrary to popular belief, the majority of these musculoskeletal injuries are not the results of accidents or sudden mishaps that break bones or strain ligaments. Rather, the type of injury referred to here usually develops gradually as a result of repeated microtrauma. Because of the slow onset and often innocuous character of the microtrauma, the condition is often ignored until the symptoms become chronic and permanent injury occurs.

Since these musculoskeletal conditions have only recently gained public attention, no uniform label or term for them has been adopted. Descriptive labels that have been used include "wear and tear" disorders, overuse injuries, osteoarthroses, and degenerative joint diseases.[7] More recently the terms repetitive motion injury, repetitive strain injury and cumulative trauma disorder (CTD) have been used to refer to those musculoskeletal impairments that appear to be work-related. CTD is used in this manual.

A useful definition of CTDs can be constructed by combining the separate meanings for each word. **Cumulative** indicates that these injuries develop gradually over periods of weeks, months, or even years as a result of repeated stresses on a particular body part. The cumulative concept is based on the theory that each repetition of an activity produces some trauma or wear and tear on the tissues and joints of the body.[8,9,10] The word **trauma** signifies bodily injury from mechanical stresses. And the term **disorders** refers to physical ailments or abnormal conditions.

CTDs belong to a collection of health problems that are considered to be work-related—that is, the disorders are more prevalent among working people than among the general population. As such, work is a risk factor for CTDs. A risk factor is any attribute, experience, or exposure that increases the probability of occurrence of a disease or disorder, though it is not necessarily a causal factor.[11]

Work may also serve as a **contributor** or **exacerbator** of an existing health problem or physical limitation. For example, work may be a factor in a disease with multiple etiologies, such as degenerative joint disease or rheumatoid arthritis. Work may also lead to an aggravation of an existing condition of non-occupational origin, such as joint pain in the elbow stemming from a previous sports-related injury. Such overuse symptoms may be experienced by weekend golfers, racket ball players and other sports participants.[12]

A worker fatigued from lack of sufficient rest, or a worker who is recovering from an illness may also be more at risk of developing a CTD than a rested or healthy worker. The risk of an overexertion injury may be further increased if the worker returns to a job requiring a level of physical exertion that exceeds his or her capacity. In general, if a sequence of events including episodes of repeated overexertion followed by insufficient recovery is repeated over successive days or weeks, a more permanent CTD will develop.

Activities associated with the onset of CTDs arise from ordinary movements that may include repetitive gripping, twisting, reaching, moving, etc. These activities, by themselves, are no more hazardous at work than at home. What makes them hazardous is chronic repetition in a forceful and awkward manner without rest or sufficient recovery time. Such conditions more often characterize work activities than leisure pursuits.

The difficulty in identifying the roles played by occupational and non-occupational factors in causing CTDs is further complicated by the role of personal factors or individual susceptibility. A worker's physical size, strength, prior injuries, and joint alignment may contribute to injury or exacerbate the adverse effects of repeated microtrauma.

Hence, CTDs are "not limited to industry or to specific occupations but to a pattern of usage."[13] Although the dynamics of repetitive and stereotypical usage still apply when non-occupational causes are suspected, the impairment occurring in a non-occupational setting is more likely to be described as an overuse injury than a CTD. If chronic, it may be regarded as the beginning stages of degenerative joint disease.[14] Regardless of the label and the origin, life activities, whether occurring in the home during leisure or at work, should be regarded as a continuum. With matters of health, there are seldom any firm boundaries that separate the work environment from the non-work environment.

The human body has great recuperative powers given the opportunity to repair itself. All that is generally needed for recovery is a sufficient interval of rest-time between episodes of high usage. When the **recovery time is insufficient**, however, and when **high repetition** is combined with **forceful** and **awkward postures, the worker is at risk of developing a CTD**.[15,16]

To illustrate and reinforce this relationship, a small pictograph was devised for each of the above key factors, illustrated in Figure 1a. Figure 1b illustrates the combined action of these factors on a worker.

Although many symptoms are associated with CTDs, the most notable are pain, restriction of joint movement, and soft tissue swelling. In the early stages there may be little or no visible signs of bruises or swollen joints. If nerves are affected, the sense of touch and manual dexterity may be reduced. Left untreated, CTDs can produce significant and lasting disability.[17,18,19]

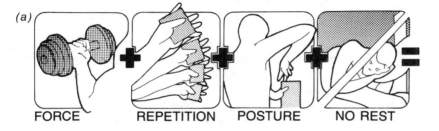

(a)

FORCE + REPETITION + POSTURE + NO REST =

CUMULATIVE TRAUMA DISORDERS

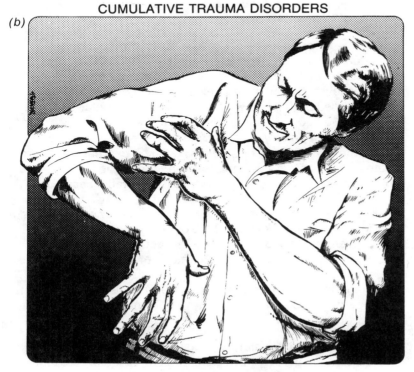

(b)

Figure 1. Four factors that account for CTDs are illustrated by the inserts at the top of the figure (a). The combination produces various degrees of discomfort and limitation of movement in the upper extremity (b).

The increase in cumulative trauma disorders

CTDs are being recognized as a leading cause of significant human suffering, loss of productivity, and economic burden on compensation systems.[20] Nowhere is this more evident than in the workplace. Just as work poses some special hazards that may result in traumatic injuries, work also poses some unique risks for incurring arthritic problems.[21]

A main reason for the evident increase in CTDs is the pace of work. Modern work is geared to production standards. The emphasis on production symbolized by the assembly line has its modern counterpart in the computerized office machine, the electronic checkout station in food stores, and the mass food processing services, to name a few examples where high-volume output is required. Most of these jobs involve performing a simple, repetitive task such as gripping, pushing, and reaching. The movement may be performed as many as 25,000 times in the course of the workday, despite physical fatigue.[22] Furthermore, during high-volume periods, minimal time exists for rest and recovery. In general, mechanization and automation have served to lighten the workload, but on the negative side it has increased the pace of work and concentrated the forces on smaller elements of the anatomy, such as the hands and wrists.[23,24]

More than half of the nation's workers now have jobs with the potential for CTDs. Major categories include construction, services, manufacturing, and clerical.[25] Data collected from the workers' compensation system revealed that the occupations of meat-cutters and butchers, miscellaneous laborers, and bottlers and canners had the largest number of claims for upper-extremity CTDs.[26]

The overall prevalence of CTDs is not known, but data collected at individual worksites suggest that CTDs are responsible for a significant amount of lost work time and high labor turnover. One of the earliest reports documented more than 60 cases during 960 worker-years of electronics assembly ($6 \cdot 4$ per 200,000 man hours worked).[27] The reported disorders included ganglionic cysts, tenosynovitis, and carpal tunnel syndrome. The severity of CTDs can also be expressed in terms of the amount of lost work and the need for medical treatments. For example, in a five-year period, 104 reportable cases of CTD were distributed among 85 employees at a plant where workers packed small parts for shipping. Nearly all of the cases required restricted duty that averaged $22 \cdot 6$ days. In addition, 11 of the most severe cases required home rest accounting for an average of $12 \cdot 6$ lost workdays. Nineteen of the affected people who failed to recover were eventually transferred to other jobs, and three people suffered permanent partial disabilities.[28] Thus, the impact of CTDs often requires significant adjustments by both workers and managers.

One reason that it is difficult to determine the true incidence of CTDs is that the person's pain and movement limitation often develops slowly over months or even years.[29] As a result, a single event or mishap cannot be identified as a cause. The chronic nature of the disorders contributes to the widespread belief that aches and pains are the inevitable price for working hard and growing old.

Today, with the proliferation of assembly-line techniques, the ever-increasing tempo of production, and the widespread use of vibrating and air-powered tools, CTDs have become a fact of modern industrial life.[30] Recent reports describe new evidence of CTDs among such diverse groups as retail clerks, computer keyboard operators, and assembly-line workers.[31] Several changes in the U.S. work force have also contributed to an increase in CTDs:

(1) An increase in service and high-tech jobs,[32]

(2) An aging workforce,[33,34] and

(3) A reduction in worker turnover.

The shift away from heavy industry and toward more **service and high-technology jobs** is exemplified by the fact that McDonald's restaurants employs more workers than U.S. Steel.[35] Though the work in these new industries may not be as physically strenuous as in the older heavy industries, it does tend to be more repetitive, prolonged, and labor intensive. The advent of robotics and increased automation has also simplified many jobs, reducing them to single repeated acts akin to the cyclic actions of machine-driven processes.

The **aging workforce** contributes to CTDs because as a person ages, the body's resilience to chronic wear and tear is reduced.[36,37] Hence a worker pays an increasingly higher health price for performing the same task as he or she grows older.

Reductions in worker turnover contribute to CTDs by reducing the flexibility of choosing less physically demanding jobs. Reduced turnover occurs during periods of high unemployment, when jobs are scarce. During economic growth there are more jobs to choose and less desirable, physically stressful jobs have higher turnover rates.

Finally, as information spreads on the causes and nature of CTDs, workers and employers are beginning to recognize that certain types of work activity can cause or contribute to these disorders. Moreover, these disorders do not have to be accepted as part of the job. Many of these disorders can be prevented.[38] Prevention is not always simple, however, since the hazard is often in the way a job is performed or how a particular tool is used.[39]

In recent years, trained professionals called ergonomists, who have special training in engineering, psychology and physiology, have made progress in redesigning tools and work stations to reduce the amount of cumulative trauma from the job. New work methods have also been devised to reduce the amount of repetition needed to perform some jobs. Examples of these workplace changes are provided in Part III of this manual.

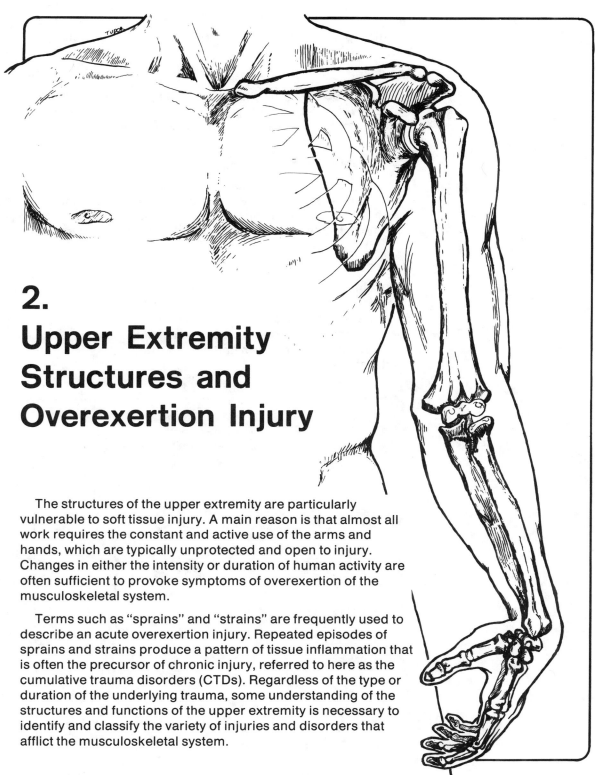

2.
Upper Extremity Structures and Overexertion Injury

The structures of the upper extremity are particularly vulnerable to soft tissue injury. A main reason is that almost all work requires the constant and active use of the arms and hands, which are typically unprotected and open to injury. Changes in either the intensity or duration of human activity are often sufficient to provoke symptoms of overexertion of the musculoskeletal system.

Terms such as "sprains" and "strains" are frequently used to describe an acute overexertion injury. Repeated episodes of sprains and strains produce a pattern of tissue inflammation that is often the precursor of chronic injury, referred to here as the cumulative trauma disorders (CTDs). Regardless of the type or duration of the underlying trauma, some understanding of the structures and functions of the upper extremity is necessary to identify and classify the variety of injuries and disorders that afflict the musculoskeletal system.

The working arm

Motion and leverage for the arms and hands are provided by ligaments and tendons at three major joints: wrist, elbow and shoulder. Together these structures form an amazingly versatile unit that allows a wide range of movement, is exceptionally strong for its size, is capable of the most delicate and precise manipulation, and alternately, is strong enough to damage itself.

Thirty-two bones make up the arm and hand. They consist of four main parts, illustrated in Figure 2, and discussed below:

Shoulder

The shoulder blade (scapula) and collar bone (clavicle) form the framework of the shoulder and serve as a pivot that allows the shoulder to be moved up, down, forward and backward.

Upper arm

The humerus is the long bone in the upper arm that is joined at the shoulder in a complex ball-and-socket joint arrangement. The shoulder joint allows an exceptionally wide range of movement, letting the arm reach out in almost every direction.

Lower arm

The ulna and radius are the two long bones in the forearm that are joined to the humerus at the elbow. The radius is the bone on the thumb side of the lower arm. Flexion and extension of the elbow occurs at the humeral-ulnar/radial joint, and supination and pronation of the forearm and hand occurs at the proximal and distal radial-ulnar joint.

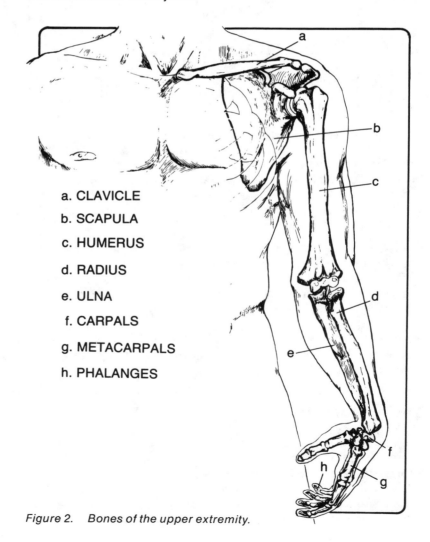

a. CLAVICLE

b. SCAPULA

c. HUMERUS

d. RADIUS

e. ULNA

f. CARPALS

g. METACARPALS

h. PHALANGES

Figure 2.   Bones of the upper extremity.

Wrist and hand with fingers

The carpals in the wrist, metacarpals in the palm, and phalanges in the fingers form the strong and flexible wrist and hand. These structures present an exceedingly complex system of pulleys and canals through which the tendons must smoothly glide to open and close the hand (Figure 3). Hand and finger movements are controlled by the muscles located in the forearm. The muscles on the back of the forearm pull the tendons that open (extend) the hand when the muscles are contracted. The muscles on the front of the forearm are connected to the fingers by tendons that run through the wrist and then through pulley-like structures on the fingers. The fingers close (flex) when these flexor muscles are contracted.[40]

Muscle and tendon injuries

Muscles are composed of thousands of tiny fibers all running in the same direction. They are red because they are filled with many blood vessels that supply them with oxygen and nutrients and carry away carbon dioxide and waste materials. Muscles can be injured in three ways. First, muscle fibers can be strained or irritated, causing temporary aching and swelling. Second, and more seriously, a small group of fibers can be torn apart. Third, a

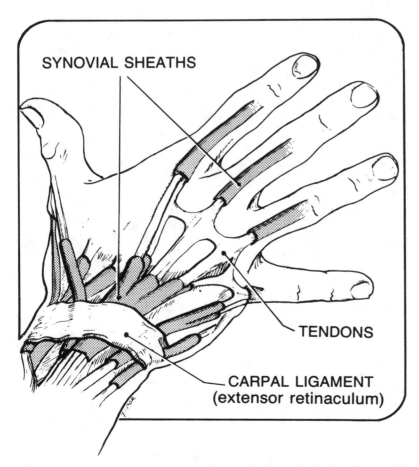

Figure 3. A pictorial view of the finger tendons, their sheaths and the carpal ligament in the hand.

muscle may be subjected to a severe blow and crushed, breaking many of its blood vessels and causing blood to seep out into a broad area. If either the blood or nerve supply to a muscle is interrupted, the muscle will get smaller and be weakened.

As Figure 4 shows, muscles are not usually attached directly to the bones; rather they are connected by **tendons** made of tough, rope-like material that is smooth, white, and shiny. Tendons do not stretch or contract—they merely transfer forces and movements from the muscles to the bones. When a joint like an elbow is severely stretched or twisted, usually in response to a sudden trauma, some tendon fibers can be torn apart like a rope that has frayed. The resulting injury is referred to as a **strain**. Scar tissue is formed that can create chronic muscle tension and is easily reinjured.

The flexor tendons of the hands pass through a rigid, 2–3 cm long tunnel in the wrist called the **carpal tunnel**. A cross sectional view of the wrist is shown in Figure 5. The tunnel walls are formed by arched carpal bones in the wrist, and its roof is formed by a tough ligament that wraps around the wrist bones.

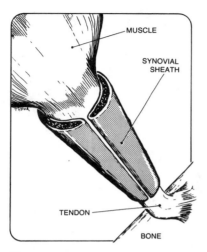

Figure 4. A magnified view of the muscle, tendon, sheath and bone.

Tendons in the wrist and hand are surrounded by a sheath containing a lubricant called synovial fluid. The tendon glides back and forth in the sheath as the muscle contracts and relaxes. A hand tendon may move as much as 5 cm in the sheath to bring a finger from a fully extended to a flexed position. With unaccustomed overuse, the lubricating fluid in the tendon sheath may be diminished causing friction between the tendon and sheath. The tendon area will feel warm, tender and painful, signaling the onset of inflammation.

Inflammation is a protective response of the surrounding tissue and blood vessels designed to limit bacterial invasion and initiate repair. Swelling and sensations of warmth occur in the injured tissue from the inflow of blood. The resulting tissue congestion distorts nerve endings that produce pain. Movement is limited as a result of increased muscle tension and muscle spasm. Moreover, repeated episodes of acute inflammation trigger the formation of extraneous fibrous tissue that is largely responsible for establishing a permanent or chronic condition. This explains why, with chronic overuse, the tendon sheath will thicken and impede tendon movement particularly in constricted areas such as the wrist.

Ligament and bursa injuries

Ligaments are strong, rope-like fibers that connect one bone to another to form a joint. Their function is to bind the bones together and limit the range of joint motion. When a joint is twisted beyond its normal range, **some fibers** of a supporting ligament may be torn or even ripped loose from the bone. This is referred to as a **sprain**. Rarely will a ligament be completely torn or ruptured unless subjected to a violent impact where a bone may also be fractured. Ligament fibers, however, that are torn from over-stretching or unaccustomed repetitive tasks contribute to permanent joint instability, which increases the risk of subsequent injury. Ligaments that are injured generally take

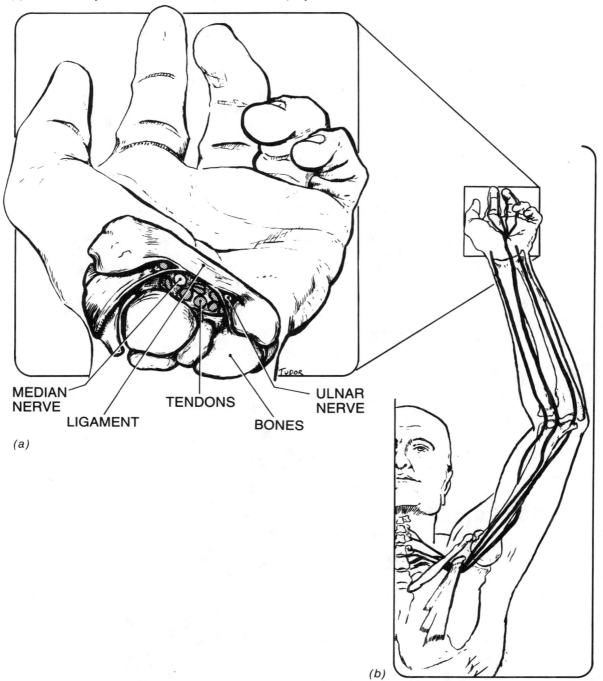

Figure 5a. *A cross section of the wrist showing the carpal tunnel that serves as a passage for finger tendons and the median nerve.*
5b. *Pathway traced by three major nerves that originate in the neck and feed into the arm and hand: ulnar, median and radial.*

weeks and even months to completely heal because of their poor blood supply.

Ligaments form a sealed **joint capsule** that encases the joint and contains a fluid that lubricates and nourishes the joint. The joint capsule functions to hold the bone ends together while allowing free movement at the joint. Ligaments reinforce the capsule at the stress points. The inner surface of the joint capsule is lined with a thin, sensitive tissue called the synovial membrane, which produces a lubricant called the synovial fluid.

Where a ligament is subject to friction, a lubricating device called a bursa shields the structure from rubbing against the bone. A **bursa** is a small, flat, fluid-filled sac lined with a synovial membrane. Bursae (plural) are located in those areas where repeated pressure is exerted during the movement of body parts such as the shoulder, elbow, and knee. Tendons in the shoulder, elbow and forearm that do have their own protective sheaths must also rely on bursae to provide a slippery cushion to reduce friction between moving parts.

One important bursa located between the shoulder tendons and the head of the humerus bone serves to cushion the rotator cuff tendons as they slide back and forth over the rough bony surface (Figure 6). Each of the shoulder bursae changes shape as the shoulder joint moves. A tendon that becomes roughened from excessive overuse or chronic use will irritate the adjacent bursa, setting up an inflammatory reaction called **bursitis**, similar to that which occurs in the tendon sheath. Bursitis inhibits the free movement of the tendon in the crowded shoulder-girdle and ultimately limits shoulder mobility.

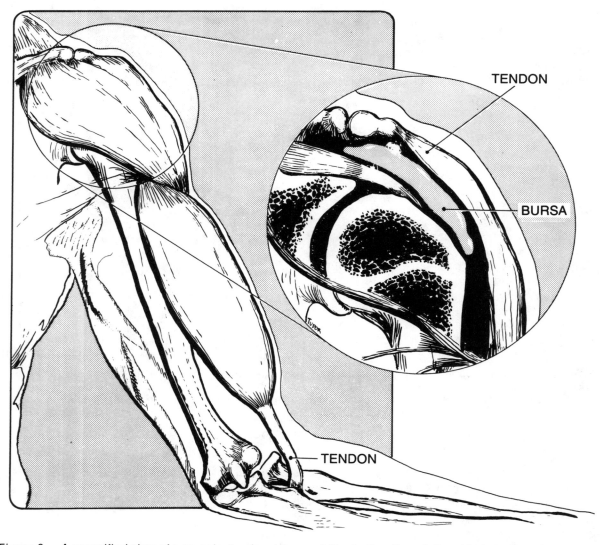

Figure 6.   A magnified view of a muscle–tendon–bone unit illustrating the relationship between a bursa and tendon in the shoulder.

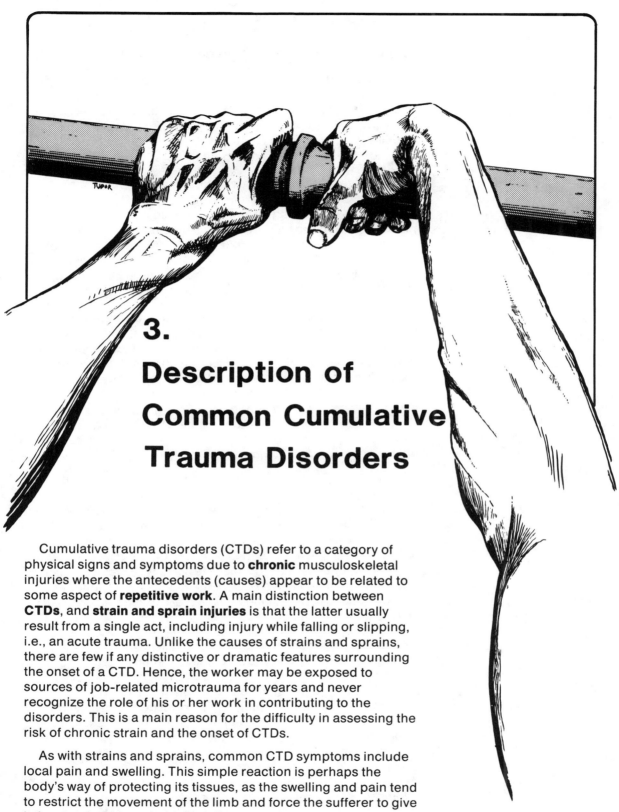

3.

Description of
Common Cumulative
Trauma Disorders

Cumulative trauma disorders (CTDs) refer to a category of physical signs and symptoms due to **chronic** musculoskeletal injuries where the antecedents (causes) appear to be related to some aspect of **repetitive work**. A main distinction between **CTDs**, and **strain and sprain injuries** is that the latter usually result from a single act, including injury while falling or slipping, i.e., an acute trauma. Unlike the causes of strains and sprains, there are few if any distinctive or dramatic features surrounding the onset of a CTD. Hence, the worker may be exposed to sources of job-related microtrauma for years and never recognize the role of his or her work in contributing to the disorders. This is a main reason for the difficulty in assessing the risk of chronic strain and the onset of CTDs.

As with strains and sprains, common CTD symptoms include local pain and swelling. This simple reaction is perhaps the body's way of protecting its tissues, as the swelling and pain tend to restrict the movement of the limb and force the sufferer to give it the rest that is needed for healing.

From an anatomical view there are three basic types of injuries to the working arm: **tendon disorder, nerve disorder or neurovascular disorder**. Several of the more frequently encountered disorders are described in this section.

Tendon disorders

Minor disorders of tendons and their sheaths are very common. Tendon disorders often occur at or near the joints where the tendons rub nearby ligaments and bones. The most frequently noted symptoms are a dull aching sensation over the tendon, discomfort with specific movements, and tenderness to touch. Seldom is there noticeable redness or local heat. Recovery is usually slow and the condition may easily become chronic if the cause is not eliminated.[41]

Tendinitis, or alternately tendonitis, is a form of tendon inflammation that occurs when a muscle/tendon unit is repeatedly tensed. With further exertion, some of the fibers that make up the tendon can actually fray or tear apart. The tendon becomes thickened, bumpy and irregular. In tendons without sheaths, such as in the shoulder, the injured area may calcify. Without rest and sufficient time for the tissues to heal, the tendon may be permanently weakened.[42]

Tenosynovitis is a general term for a repetitive-induced tendon injury involving the synovial sheath. With extreme repetition, the sheath will be stimulated to produce excessive amounts of synovial fluid. The excess fluid accumulates and the sheath becomes swollen and painful. For example, repetitions that exceed 1500 to 2000 per hour are known to produce identifiable symptoms of tendon sheath irritation in the hands.[43] According to Dorland's Illustrated Medical Dictionary, the names tendosynovitis, tendovaginitis, tenovaginitis, and peritendinitis are synonymous with tenosynovitis.[44]

If the tendon surface becomes irritated and rough, and if the sheath becomes inflamed and continues to press on the tendon, a condition called **stenosing tenosynovitis** may be diagnosed.[45] Stenosis refers to a progressive constriction of the tendon sheath. **De Quervain's disease**, named after the French physician who first described it, is the most recognized stenosing tenosynovitis. This disorder affects the tendons on the side of the wrist and at the base of the thumb. These tendons are connected to muscles on the back of the forearm that contract to pull the thumb back and away from the hand.[46]

De Quervain's disease is attributed to excessive friction between two thumb tendons and their common sheath. The repetitive friction accounts for the abnormal thickening of the fibrous sheath and resultant constriction of the tendons. Combinations of hand twisting and forceful gripping, similar to a clothes-wringing movement, will place sufficient stress on the tendons to cause De Quervain's disorders.[47] In general, the flexor tendons and sheaths on the palmar surface of the hand are the most common sites for CTDs.

If the tendon sheath of a finger is sufficiently swollen so that the tendon becomes locked in the sheath, attempts to move that finger will cause a snapping and jerking movements, a condition called **stenosing tenosynovitis crepitans** or **trigger finger**.[48] The palm side of the fingers is the usual site for trigger finger. This disorder is often associated with using tools that have handles with hard or sharp edges.[49]

A **ganglionic cyst** is yet another form that a tendon sheath disorder may take. The affected sheath swells up with synovial fluid and causes a bump under the skin, often on the wrist. An illustration of a ganglion cyst on the wrist is shown in Figure 7.[50] At one time ganglions were called Bible bumps because the Bible (then the most available book), was used to pound and rupture the ganglion. Today, ganglions are treated surgically.[51]

Unsheathed tendons are found in the elbow and shoulder joints. The elbow is particularly vulnerable to tendinitis because of the imbalance between the large forearm muscles and the small insertion area on the epicondyle of the humerus bone (elbow). The finger extensor muscles that are attached to the elbow control the movement of the wrist and hand. When strained or subjected to overuse, the tendons become irritated and radiate pain from the elbow down the forearm, a condition referred to as lateral epicondylitis (Figure 8).[52] Activities that trigger the condition are associated with the use of the arm for impact or jerky throwing motions, hence the terms "**tennis elbow**, pitcher's and bowler's elbow." Symptoms are most common on the outer side of the elbow.

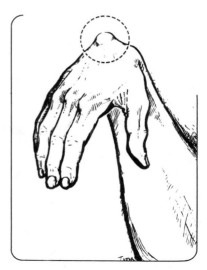

Figure 7. *A ganglionic cyst on the wrist.*

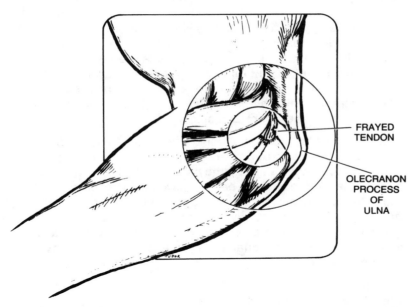

FRAYED
TENDON

OLECRANON
PROCESS
OF
ULNA

Figure 8. *Close-up view of tendons involved in tennis elbow (lateral epicondylitis).*

Golfer's elbow (medial epicondylitis) is an irritation of the tendon attachments of the finger flexor muscles on the inside of the elbow. Epicondylitis is associated with tasks that require repeated or forceful rotation of the forearm and bending of the wrist at the same time.[53] These injuries earned their names because they can afflict athletes, but the vast majority of people who suffer with epicondylitis have never picked up a racket or golf club.

The most common shoulder tendon disorder is **rotator cuff tendinitis**. Other names or descriptions for this type of disorder include: supraspinatus tendinitis, subdeltoid bursitis, subacromial bursitis, and partial tear of rotator cuff. The rotator cuff consists of four tendons that fuse over the joint to provide a main source of stability and mobility for the shoulder. The rotator cuff tendons rotate the arm inward and outward and assist in moving the arm away from the side. In performing this motion the rotator cuff tendons pass through a small bony passage between the humerus and an overhanging bony process, the acromion. A bursa serves as a cushion to protect the tendons from the bony ridge.

Shoulder disorders are often associated with work that requires the elbow to be in an elevated position that puts stress on the shoulder tendons and bursae.[54,55] The wear and tear of repeated overhead motions contributes to the thickening of both tendons and bursa, which can give rise to the "frozen shoulder" syndrome, characterized by severe pain and functional impairment. The shoulder is also a frequent target for degenerative joint disease and rheumatoid arthritis.

Nerve disorders

Nerve CTDs occur when repeated or sustained work activities expose the nerves to pressure from hard, sharp edges of the work surface, tools, or nearby bones, ligaments, and tendons.[56] For example, a seated worker may support his arm and shoulder by leaning the forearm against the hard edge of a work bench. In this position, pressure is placed on the ulnar nerve as it passes over the elbow. In time, numbness and tingling may result over and below the little finger—much like the sensation produced when a person bumps his "funny bone." This condition used to be called telephone-operator's elbow.[57]

The tendons for flexing the fingers, the median nerve and blood vessels pass through the carpal tunnel, under the carpal ligament, from the forearm to the hand.[58] (See Figures 4 and 5.) If any of the tendon sheaths become swollen in the cramped carpal tunnel, the median nerve may be pinched. This is one of the causes of an increasingly common CTD, the **carpal tunnel syndrome**.[59] Other terms used to describe this disorder include writer's cramp, occupational neuritis, partial thenar atrophy and median neuritis.

Pressure on, or compression of, the median nerve can occur from chronic irritation and swelling (tenosynovitis) of the finger flexor tendons inside the wrist. The pressure interferes with normal sensations felt on the palm and back areas of the hand. Several specific positions, movements, and hand grips may also be responsible for the onset of carpal tunnel syndrome.[60] Jobs that combine high force and high repetition pose the greatest risk.[61]

Symptoms of carpal tunnel syndrome include pain, numbness, and tingling of the hands. These sensations usually are felt in the areas of the skin connected to the median nerve—the first three fingers and the base of the thumb. The condition may affect both hands (bilateral) or only the dominant hand.[62] Affected areas of the hand are illustrated by the shaded area in Figure 9. Symptoms are often most acute while sleeping. Advanced cases may include a wasting away of the thenar muscles at the base of the thumb and an apparent weakness and clumsiness of the hand.[63]

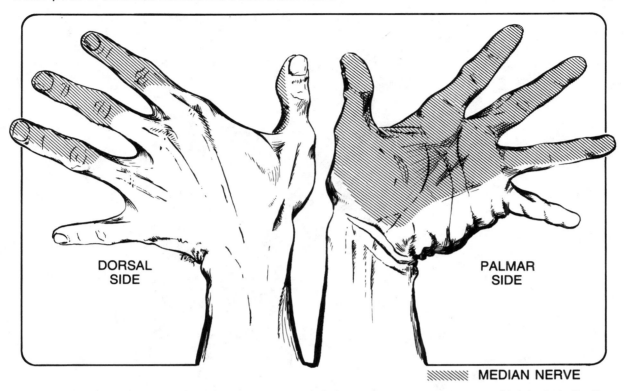

DORSAL SIDE

PALMAR SIDE

▨▨▨ **MEDIAN NERVE**

Figure 9. Shaded areas typically affected by symptoms of carpal tunnel syndrome, which include tingling, numbness, and pain.

Neurovascular disorders

Some CTDs involve both the nerves and adjacent blood vessels. One of the most common conditions of this type is the **thoracic outlet syndrome**, which involves the shoulder and upper arm.[64] Thoracic outlet syndrome is a general term for compression of the nerves and blood vessels between the neck and shoulder. Other terms such as neurovascular compression syndrome, hyperabduction syndrome, cervicobrachial disorder, brachial plexus neuritis, and costoclavicular syndrome are also used depending on the exact location of the condition. The symptoms of thoracic outlet syndrome are similar to those of carpal tunnel syndrome, namely numbness in the fingers of the hand. The arm may feel as if it is "going to sleep," and the pulse at the wrist may be weakened.[65] The major symptoms are due to the compression of nerves and blood vessels between the neck and the shoulder—the neurovascular bundle (Figure 10).

The neurovascular bundle, also referred to as the brachial plexus, consists of a network of large arteries and veins found under the coracoid process, which provides blood circulation for the arm. If the circulation is impeded by activities or postures that put excessive pressure on these blood vessels, the adjacent tendons, ligaments and muscles are deprived of oxygen and nutrients. This produces an ischemic condition, which slows muscle recovery and limits the duration of muscle activity. Certain chronic diseases and congenital defects produce similar effects, such as arteriosclerosis, cervical rib or abnormal muscles.[66] In a work situation, these blood vessels are compressed as a result of various activities or postures that include: pulling the shoulders back and down, as a soldier does when he stands at attention, or as a person does when carrying a stretcher, knapsack, or suitcase, or when the work requires frequent reaching above shoulder level (Figure 10).[67]

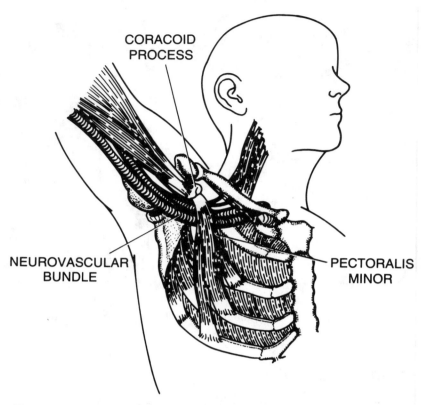

CORACOID
PROCESS

NEUROVASCULAR
BUNDLE

PECTORALIS
MINOR

Figure 10.   Abduction, moving the elbow away from the body, causes the neurovascular bundle to be stretched under the pectoralis muscle, much like a belt stretched around a pulley.

Vibration syndrome is also referred to as white finger or Raynaud's phenomenon. Occupational vibration syndrome is characterized by recurrent episodes of finger blanching due to complete closure of the digital arteries. Exposure to cold may serve to trigger vasospasm in the fingers. The condition is caused in part by forceful gripping and prolonged use of vibrating tools, such as pneumatic hammers, chain saws, and power grinders. Common symptoms include intermittent numbness and tingling in the fingers; skin that turns pale, ashen, and cold; and eventual loss of sensation and control in the fingers and hands.[68,69]

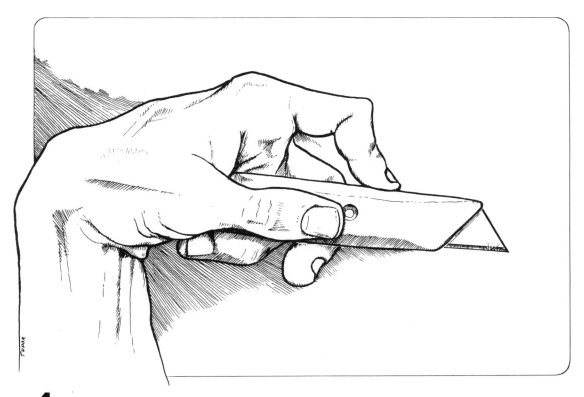

4.

Jobs and Cumulative Trauma Disorders

Types of jobs implicated

Upper extremity CTDs have been asociated with work activity in a variety of industries, jobs, and specific tasks. Many of the reports are clinical case studies from medical journals. Others involve evaluations of specific types of jobs where workers exhibited evidence of CTDs. Table 1 is an initial compilation of such information. It is by no means exhaustive, as there has been no systematic survey of all industries and jobs to define such risk factors. Occupational factors that have been noted as causing or aggravating the disorder have also been listed.

Problems with posture, force and repetition

The majority of the occupational factors noted in Table 1 can be categorized as involving one or more of the following components: awkward **postures** of the wrist or shoulders, excessive manual **force**, and high rates of manual **repetition**. For example, even mechanical stresses on hand tissue, a common CTD in heavy manual work, can be traced to combinations of forceful gripping and repetitive pounding with hands.

Table 1.   Job, identified disorder, and occupational risk factors

Type of job	Disorder	Occupational factors
1. Buffing/grinding	Tenosynovitis Thoracic outlet Carpal tunnel De Quervain's Pronator teres	Repetitive wrist motions, prolonged flexed shoulders, vibration, forceful ulnar deviation, repetitive forearm pronation.
2. Punch press operators	Tendinitis of wrist and shoulder De Quervain's	Repetitive forceful wrist extension/flexion, repetitive shoulder abduction/flexion, forearm supination. Repetitive ulnar deviation in pushing controls.
3. Overhead assembly (welders, painters, auto repair)	Thoracic outlet Shoulder tendinitis	Sustained hyperextension of arms. Hands above shoulders.
4. Belt conveyor assembly	Tendinitis of shoulder and wrist Carpal tunnel Thoracic outlet	Arms extended, abducted, or flexed more than 60 degrees, repetitive, forceful wrist motions.
5. Typing, keypunch, cashier	Tension neck Thoracic outlet Carpal tunnel	Static, restricted posture, arms abducted/flexed high speed finger movement, palmar base pressure, ulnar deviation.
6. Sewers and cutters	Thoracic outlet De Quervain's Carpal tunnel	Repetitive shoulder flexion, repetitive ulnar deviation. Repetitive wrist flexion/extension, palmar base pressure.
7. Small parts assembly (wiring, bandage wrap)	Tension neck Thoracic outlet Wrist tendinitis Epicondylitis	Prolonged restricted posture, forceful ulnar deviation and thumb pressure, repetitive wrist motion, forceful wrist extension and pronation.
8. Musicians	Wrist tendinitis Carpal tunnel Epicondylitis Thoracic outlet	Repetitive forceful wrist motions, palmar base pressure, prolonged shoulder abduction/flexion, forceful wrist extension with forearm pronation.
9. Bench work (glass cutters, phone operators)	Ulnar nerve entrapment	Sustained elbow flexion with pressure on ulnar groove.
10. Operating room personnel	Thoracic outlet Carpal tunnel De Quervain's	Prolonged shoulder flexion, repetitive wrist flexion, ulnar deviation (holding retractors).
11. Packing	Tendinitis of shoulder and wrist Tension neck Carpal tunnel De Quervain's	Prolonged load on shoulders, repetitive wrist motions, over-exertion, forceful ulnar deviation.
12. Truck driver	Thoracic outlet	Prolonged shoulder abduction and flexion.
13. Core making	Tendinitis of the wrist	Repetitive wrist motions.
14. Housekeeping, cooks	De Quervain's Carpal tunnel	Scrubbing, washing, rapid wrist rotational movements.
15. Carpenters, bricklayers	Carpal tunnel Guyon tunnel	Hammering, pressure on palmar base.
16. Stockroom, shipping	Thoracic outlet Shoulder-tendinitis	Reaching overhead. Prolonged load on shoulder in unnatural position.
17. Material handling	Thoracic outlet Shoulder-tendinitis	Carrying heavy load on shoulders.
18. Lumber/construction	Shoulder-tendinitis Epicondylitis	Repetitive throwing of heavy load.
19. Butcher/meat packing	De Quervain's Carpal tunnel	Ulnar deviation, flexed wrist with exertion.
20. Letter carriers	Shoulder problems Thoracic outlet	Carrying heavy load with shoulder strap.

Posture

Certain jobs require the worker to assume a variety of awkward postures that pose significant biomechanical stress to the joints of the upper extremity and surrounding soft tissues. Research has established that posture is a significant factor in the development of CTDs.[70] Awkward postures include any fixed or constrained body position. Other postures considered undesirable include those that: (1) overload the muscles and tendons, (2) load joints in an uneven or asymmetrical manner, or (3) involve a static load on the musculature.[71]

CTDs that have been identified include tenosynovitis of the flexors and extensors of the forearm and CTS arising from extreme flexion and extension of the wrist.[72,73] Ulnar and radial deviations of the wrist are associated with De Quervain's disease.[74] Various shoulder ailments, including thoracic outlet syndrome, have been associated with jobs that require workers to reach behind or above their shoulder level repeatedly[75,76] Shoulder disorders are also associated with reaching down and behind the torso.[77] Extreme flexion of the elbow is associated with cubital tunnel syndrome.[78] Extreme rotation of the forearm is associated with medial and lateral epicondylitis.[79,80]

Force

The force required to perform various occupational activities is also a critical factor in contributing to the onset of CTDs.[81,82] The load or the pressure put on various tissues of the body can easily amount to hundreds of pounds. As the muscle effort increases in response to high task load, circulation to the muscle decreases causing more rapid muscle fatigue. Recovery time can exceed actual work time for jobs where force requirements are high. Deprived of sufficient recovery time, soft tissue injuries will occur. Obviously, bones will break and skin and muscles will tear if the strain is too great. What is not as obvious is the mechanical stresses on the tendons and nerves produced by contact with sharp edges of hard objects that are held in the hand.

Scissors, for example, that rub on the sides of the fingers may also cause compression of the digital nerves in the fingers.[83,84] Manual forces are transmitted through the skin to underlying tendons. The palmar side of the fingers is a common site of stenosing tenosynovitis crepitans (trigger finger).[85] Trigger finger is associated with forceful gripping of tools that have hard or sharp edges on their handles. Workers performing tasks where force is applied with the wrist in a laid back or dorsiflexion posture, such as in pushing, increase their risk of developing an entrapment of the ulnar nerve where it passes under the hamate bone in the wrist (Guyon canal). A case was reported where a worker used the fleshy part of his palm to force wood through a powersaw.[86]

Mechanical stress produced by vibrating tools such as power sanders may also contribute to the development of a vibration syndrome that affects the fingers. The vibration causes constriction of blood vessels, which if chronic, may damage nerves in the fingers. Common descriptive terms for this syndrome include: "white finger, and occupational Raynaud's." Mechanical stresses are also produced by pounding with the hand. In general, acceptable limits of force on various parts of the body are conditioned by many variables. Age, sex, body build and general health all help determine the amount of force that is tolerable.[87]

Repetition

Jobs that require the worker to perform highly repetitive motions also contribute to the onset of CTDs.[88] Specifically, the more repetitive the task, the more rapid and frequent are the muscle contractions. Muscles required to contract at a high velocity develop less tension than when contracting at a slower velocity for the same load. Hence, tasks requiring high rates of repetition require more muscle effort, and consequently more time for recovery, than less repetitive tasks. In this manner tasks with high repetition rates can become sources of trauma even when the required forces are minimal and normally safe.[89]

Carpal tunnel syndrome, for example, appears to be induced more by the repetitiveness of the task than by the force levels.[90] Findings from another study on repetition indicated that the prevalence of tenosynovitis and humeral tendinitis is significantly higher for workers engaged in machine-paced assembly work than for shop assistants with variable tasks. Repetitive motions of the hands for some assembly-line workers in the study reached 25,000 cycles per workday.[91] In general, the speed, intensity, and work pace typical of modern industry has been proved debilitating to many millions of workers.[92] Researchers are just beginning to assess the acceptable or safe limits of repetition.

Non-occupational factors associated with CTDs

Occupational activities may be only partially responsible for the development of disorders associated with repetitive trauma. Non-occupational activites that stress the musculoskeletal system can produce the same types of disorders.[93]

Athletic activities such as racket sports and throwing have been associated with the development of tendinitis, tenosynovitis, degenerative joint disease, and peripheral nerve entrapments. Hobbies such as knitting, sewing, or the playing of musical instruments have also been associated with the development of these disorders.[94] Traumatic accidents that result in fractures of the bones of the upper extremities may predispose a person to many of the disorders that are discussed in this manual.[95] Various systemic diseases or conditions may also predispose a person to many of the common CTDs. Examples include: rheumatoid arthritis, hypertension, diabetes, thyroid disorders, kidney disorders, gout, alcoholism, pregnancy, use of oral contraceptives, and gynecological surgery and disorders.[96,97]

Sometimes it is difficult to clearly distinguish occupational CTDs from non-occupational conditions. In such cases it may be necessary to closely monitor the working conditions and review all the symptoms reported by other workers doing a similar job. Although the finding that co-workers doing similar jobs do not experience symptoms of CTDs, it does not preclude an occupational basis for the condition due to differences in individual susceptibility and work history. In general, to control these disorders effectively, the key risk factors should be identified before any corrective actions are implemented. Furthermore, by controlling occupational stresses that cause CTDs, and by counseling employees on non-occupational factors, the frequency of these work-related disorders can be reduced.[98]

References—Part I

1. Ramazinni, B., 1717 and 1940, In W. Wright (trans.): *The Disease of Workers*, (Chicago: University of Chicago Press).

2. Hunter, D., 1978, *The Diseases of Occupations*, 6th edition, (London: Hodder and Stoughton), pp. 857–864.

3. U.S. Department of Labor, Bureau of Labor Statistics, 1984, *Occupational Injuries and Illnesses in the United States by Industry, 1982*. Bulletin 2196, pp. 2–3.

4. Putz-Anderson, V., Pizatella, T. and Tanaka, S., 1986, *A Proposed National Strategy for the Prevention of Musculoskeletal Injuries*. National Institute for Occupational Safety and Health and Associations of Schools of Public Health, pp. 17–34. [NTIS 87 114 740]

5. Kelsey, J.L., 1982, *Epidemiology of Musculoskeletal Disorders*, (New York: Oxford Press) p. 7.

6. Haber, L.D., 1971, Disabling effects of chronic disease and impairment. *J. Chron. Dis.*, **24**, 469–487.

7. Salter, R.B., 1970, *Textbook of Disorders and Injuries of the Musculoskeletal System*, (Baltimore, MD: Williams & Wilkins) pp. 194–195.

8. Radin, E.L., 1976, Mechanical aspects of osteoarthrosis. *Bulletin on the Rheum. Diseases*, **26**:7, 862–865.

9. Pugh, J., 1982, Biomechanical aspects of osteoarthritic joints, mechanisms and noninvasive detection. In: *Osteoarthromechanics*, edited by D.N. Ghista, (New York: McGraw-Hill) p. 162.

10. Cailliet, R., 1977, *Soft Tissue Pain and Disability*, (Philadelphia: F.A. Davis Co.) pp. 23–24.

11. Last, J.M., 1983, *Dictionary of Epidemiology*, (New York: Oxford University Press) p. 93.

12. Benjamin, B.E. and Borden, G., 1984, *Listen To Your Pain*, (London: Penguin Books) pp. 20–24.

13. Williams, H.J., and Ward, J.R., 1983, Musculoskeletal Occupational Syndromes. In: *Environmental and Occupational Medicine*, edited by W.N. Rom, A.D. Renzetti, Jr., J.S. Lee, and V.E. Archer, (Boston: Little, Brown and Co.) p. 351.

14. Hadler, N.M., Gillings, D.B., Imbus, H.R., Levitin, P.M., Makuc, D., Utsinger, P.D., Yount, W.J., Slusser, D. and Moskovitz, N., 1978, Hand structure and function in an industrial setting: Influence of three patterns of stereotyped, repetitive usage. *Arthritis and Rheumatism*, **21**(2) 210–220.

15. Silverstein, B.A., Fine, L.J. and Armstrong, T.J., 1986, Hand

wrist cumulative trauma disorders in industry. *Br. J. of Ind. Med.*, **43,** 779–784.

16. Feldman, R.G., Goldman, R. and Keyserling, W.M., 1983, Peripheral nerve entrapment syndromes and ergonomic factors. *Am. J. Ind. Med.*, **4,** 661–681.

17. Kelly, A.P. and Jacobson, H.S., 1964, Hand disability due to tenosynovitis. *Ind. Med. and Surg.*, **33,** 570–574.

18. Thompson, A.R., Plewes, L.W. and Shaw, E.G., 1951, Peritendinitis crepitans and simple tenosynovitis: A clinical study of 544 cases in industry. *Brit. J. of Ind. Med.*, **8,** 150–160.

19. Rowe, M.L., 1985, *Orthopaedic Problems at Work*, (New York: Perinton Press) pp. 1–7.

20. Kelsey, J.L., White, A.A., Pastides H. and Bisbee, Jr., G.E., 1979, The impact of musculoskeletal disorders on the population of the U.S. *J. of Bone and Joint Surg.*, **61**A(7), 959–963.

21. Anderson, J.A.D., 1984, Arthrosis and its relation to work. *Scand. J. Work Environ. and Health*, **10,** 429–433.

22. Luopajarvi, T., Kuorinka, I., Virolainen, M. and Holmberg, M., 1979, Prevalence of tenosynovitis and other injuries of the upper extremities in repetitive work. *Scand. J. Work Environ. and Health*, **5**(3), 48–55.

23. Ohara, H., Nakagiri, S., Itani, T., Wake, K. and Aoyama, H., 1976, Occupational health hazards resulting from elevated work rate situations. *J. Human Ergol.* **5,** 173–182.

24. Kuorinka, I. and Koskinen, P., 1979, Occupational rheumatic diseases and upper limb strain in manual jobs in a light mechanical industry. *Scand. J. Work Environ. and Health,* **5**(3), 39–47.

25. U.S. Department of Commerce, Bureau of Industrial Economics, 1984, *U.S. Industrial Outlook: Prospects for over 3000 Industries,* 25th edition (Washington, DC).

26. Jenson, R.C., Klein, B.P. and Sanderson, L.M., 1983, Motion-related wrist disorders traced to industries, occupational groups. *Monthly Labor Review.* pp. 13–16.

27. Hymovich, L. and Lindholm, M., 1966, Hand, wrist, and forearm injuries: the result of repetitive motions. *J. Occup. Med.,* **8**(11), 573–577.

28. Wisseman, C. and Badger, D., 1977, *Hazard Evaluation and Technical Assistance, Report* No. TA 76–93, USDHEW, CDC, NIOSH, Cincinnati, Ohio.

29. Bjelle, A., Hagberg, M. and Michaelsson, G., 1979, Clinical and ergonomic factors in prolonged shoulder pain among industrial workers. *Scand. J. Work Environ. and Health,* **5,** 205–210.

30. Habes, D.J. and Putz-Anderson, V., 1985, The NIOSH program for evaluating biomechanical hazards in the workplace. *J. of Safety Research,* **16**(2), 49–60.

31. Sallstrom, J. and Schmidt, H., 1984, Cervicobrachial disorders in certain occupations, with special reference to compression in the thoracic outlet. *Am. J. of Ind. Med.,* **6,** 45–52.

32. Scott, J.W., 1982, The mechanization of women's work. *Scientific American,* **247**(3), 167–187.

33. Donnedly, H., 1981, Percentage of aged to grow rapidly. . . *Congressional Quarterly,* pp. 2330–2332.

34. Cunningham, L.S. and Kelsey, J.L. Epidemiology of musculoskeletal impairments and associated disability. *Am. J. Pub. Health,* **74**(6), 574–579.

35. "Golden arches not blast furnaces symbolize the current economy", 1981, *Newsweek,* Feb 16.

36. Hansson, T. and Roos, B., 1981, The relation between bone mineral content, experimental compression fractures, and disc degeneration in lumbar vertebrae. *Spine,* **6,** 147–153.

37. Muckart, R.D., 1964, Stenosing tendovaginitis of abductor pollicis longus and extensor pollicis brevis at the radial styloid (de Quervain's disease). *Clin. Orthop. and Related Res.,* **33,** 201–208.

38. McKenzie, F., Storment, J., Van Hook, P. and Armstrong, T.J., 1985, A program for control of repetitive trauma disorders associated with hand tool operations in a telecommunications manufacturing facility. *Am. Ind. Hyg. Assoc. J.,* **46**(11), 674–678.

39. Tichauer, E.R. and Gage, H., 1977, Ergonomic principles basic to hand tool design. *Am. Ind. Hyg. Assoc. J.,* **38,** 622–634.

40. Napier, J.R., 1980, *Hands,* (New York: Pantheon Books) pp. 60–66.

41. Lipscomb, P.R., 1959, Tenosynovitis of the hand and the wrist: Carpal tunnel syndrome, De Quervain's disease, trigger digit. *Clinical Orthop.,* **13,** 164–181.

42. Curwin, S. and Stanish, W.D., 1984, *Tendinitis: Its Etiology and Treatment.* (Lexington: Collamore Press) pp. 25–36.

43. Hammer, A.W., 1934, Tenosynovitis, *Medical Record,* **140,** 353–355.

44. *Dorland's Illustrated Medical Dictionary,* 1974, (25th ed.) (Philadelphia, PA: W.B. Saunders, Co) pp. 1131–1515.

45. Kelly, A.P. and Jacobson, H.S., 1964, Hand disability due to tenosynovitis. *Ind. Med. and Surg.,* **33,** 570–574.

46. Pick, R.Y., 1979, De Quervain's disease: a clinical triad. *Clin. Orthop. Rel. Res.,* **143,** 165–166.

47. Lamphier, T.A., Crooker, C. and Crooker, J.L., 1965, De Quervain's disease. *Ind. Med. and Surg.,* **34,** 847–856.

48. Younghusband, O.Z. and Black, J.D., 1963, De Quervain's Disease: Stenosing Tenovaginitis at the radial styloid process. *Can. Med. Assoc. J.,* **89,** 508–512.

49. Thompson, A.R., Plewes, L.W. and Shaw, E.G., 1951, Peritendinitis crepitans and simple tenosynovitis: a clinical study of 544 cases in industry. *Br. J. Ind. Med.,* **8,** 150–160.

50. De Orsay, R.H., Mecray, Jr. P.M. and Ferguson, L.K., 1937, Pathology and treatment of ganglion. *Am. J. Surg.,* **36**(1), 313–319.

51. Burt, T.B., MacCarter, D.K., Gelman, M.I. and Samuelson, C.O., 1980, Clinical manifestations of synovial cysts. *West. J. Med.,* **133**(2), 99–104.

52. Boyd, H.B. and McLeod, Jr. A.C., 1973, Tennis elbow. *J. Bone Joint Surg.,* **55A**(6), 1183–1187.

53. Murley, A.G.H., 1975, The painful elbow. *Practitioner,* **215,** 36–41.

54. Bateman, J.E., 1968, Neurovascular syndromes related to the clavicle. *Clin. Orthop. Rel. Res.,* **58,** 75–82.

55. Bateman, J.E., 1983, Neurologic painful conditions affecting the shoulder. *Clin. Orthop. Rel. Res.,* **173,** 44–54.

56. Feldman, R.G., Goldman, R. and Keyserling, W.M., 1983, Peripheral nerve entrapment syndromes and ergonomic factors. *Am. J. Ind. Med., 4,* 661–681.
57. Armstrong, T.J., 1983, *An Ergonomics Guide to Carpal Tunnel Syndrome.* American Industrial Hygiene Association, Akron.
58. Tanzer, R.C., 1959, The carpal tunnel syndrome. *J. Bone Joint Surg., 41*(a), 626–634.
59. Phalen, G.S., 1972, The carpal tunnel syndrome, clinical evaluation of 598 hands. *Clin. Orthop. Rel. Res., 83,* 29–40.
60. Smith, E.M., Sonstegard, D.A. and Anderson, Jr., W.H., 1977, Carpal tunnel syndrome: contribution of flexor tendons. *Arch. Phys. Med. Rehabil., 58,* 379–385.
61. Silverstein, B.A., Fine, L.J. and Armstrong, T.J., 1987, Occupational factors and carpal tunnel syndrome. *Am. J. Ind. Med., 11,* 343–358.
62. Reinstein, L., 1981, Hand dominance in carpal tunnel syndrome. *Arch. Phys. Med. Rehabil., 62,* 202–203.
63. Phalen, G.S., 1966, The carpal tunnel syndrome. *J. Bone Joint Surg., 48A*(2), 211–228.
64. Bateman, J.E., 1968, Neurovascular syndromes related to the clavicle. *Clin. Ortho. Rel. Res., 58,* 75–82.
65. Tyson, R.R. and Kaplan, G.F., 1975, Modern concepts of diagnosis and treatment of the thoracic outlet syndrome. *Orthop. Clinics of North America, 6,* 507–519.
66. Dale, W.A., 1982, Thoracic outlet compression syndrome. *Arch. Surg., 117,* 1437–1445.
67. Beyer, J.A. and Wright, I.S., 1951, Hyperabduction syndrome, with special reference to its relationship to Raynaud's syndrome. *Circulation, 4,* 161–172.
68. National Institute for Occupational Safety and Health, 1983, *Current Intelligence Bulletin. No. 38 Vibration syndrome.* DHHS (NIOSH) Pub. No. 83–110.
69. Bovenzi, M., 1986, Some pathophysiological aspects of vibration-induced white finger. *Eur. J. Appl. Physiol., 55,* 381–389.
70. Armstrong, T.J., 1985, Upper extremity posture: Definition, measurement and control. *Proceedings of the International Occupational Ergonomics Symposium.* Zadar, Yugoslavia.
71. Van Wely, P., 1970, Design and disease. *Applied Ergonomics, 1*(5), 262–269.
72. Smith, E.M., Sonstegard, D.A. and Anderson, Jr., W.H., 1977, Carpal tunnel syndrome: contribution of flexor tendons. *Arch. Phys. Med. Rehabil., 58,* 379–385.
73. Armstrong, T.J. and Chaffin, D.B., 1979, Carpal tunnel syndrome and selected personal attributes. *J. Occup. Med., 21*(7), 481–486.
74. Muckart, R.D., 1964, Stenosing tendovaginitis of abductor pollicis longus and extensor pollicis brevis at the radial styloid (De Quervain's Disease) *Clin. Orthop. Rel. Res., 33,* 201–208.
75. Hagberg, M., 1984, Occupational musculoskeletal stress and disorders of the neck and shoulder: a review of possible pathophysiology. *Int. Arch. Occup. Environ. Health, 53,* 269–278.
76. Bjelle, A., Hagberg, M. and Michaelsson, G., 1979, Clinical and ergonomic factors in prolonged shoulder pain among industrial workers. *Scand. J. Work Environ. and Health, 5,* 205–210.

77. Nichols, H.M., 1967, Anatomic structures of the thoracic outlet. *Clin. Orthop. Rel. Res.,* **51,** 17–25.

78. Feldman, R.G., Goldman, R. and Keyserling, W.M., 1983, Peripheral nerve entrapment syndromes and ergonomic factors. *Am. J. Ind. Med.,* **4,** 661–681.

79. Tichauer, E.R., 1976, Biomechanics sustains occupational safety and health. *Ind. Engin.,* **8,** 16–56.

80. Gardner, R.C., 1970, Tennis elbow: diagnosis, pathology and treatment. *Clin. Orthop.,* **72,** 248–253.

81. Silverstein, B.A., Fine, L.J. and Armstrong, T.J., 1986, Hand wrist cumulative trauma disorders in industry. *Brit. J. Ind. Med.,* **43,** 779–784.

82. Armstrong, T.J., Foulke, J.A., Joseph, B.S. and Goldstein, S.A., 1982, Investigation of cumulative trauma disorders in a poultry processing plant. *Am. Ind. Hyg. Assoc. J.,* **43**(2), 103–116.

83. Greenberg, L. and Chaffin, D.B., 1977, *Workers and Their Tools,* (Midland, Michigan: Pendell Publishing Co.) pp. 63–65.

84. Dobyns, J.H., O'Brien, E.T. and Linscheid, R.L., 1972, Bowler's thumb: Diagnosis and treatment. *J. Bone Joint Surg.,* **54**(A), 751–755.

85. Quinnell, R.C., 1980, Conservative management of trigger finger. *Practitioner,* **224,** 187–190.

86. Swanson, A.B., Biddulph, S.L., Baughman, Jr., F.A. and de Groot, G., 1972, Ulnar nerve compression due to an anomalous muscle in the Canal of Guyon. *Clin. Orthop. and Rel. Res.,* **83,** 64–69.

87. Armstrong, T.J., 1986, Ergonomics and cumulative trauma disorders. *Hand Clinics,* **2**(3), 553–565.

88. Hymovich, L. and Lindholm, M., 1966, Hand, wrist, and forearm injuries: the result of repetitive motions. *J. Occup. Med.,* **8**(11), 573–577.

89. Kaplan, P.E., 1983, Carpal tunnel syndrome in typists. *JAMA,* **250**(6), 821–822.

90. Armstrong, T.J., Fine, L.J. and Silverstein, B.A., 1985, *Occupational Risk Factors. Final Contract Report* to NIOSH No. 200–82–2507. Cincinnati, Ohio.

91. Luopajarvi, T., Kuorinka, I., Virolainen, M. and Holmberg, M., 1979, Prevalence of tenosynovitis and other injuries of the upper extremities in repetitive work. *Scand. J. Work Environ. and Health,* **5**(3), 48–55.

92. Ohara, H., Nakagiri, S., Itani, T., Wake, K. and Aoyama, H., 1976, Occupational health hazards resulting from elevated work rate situations. *J. Human Ergol.,* **5,** 173–182.

93. Cannon, L.J., Bernacki, E.J. and Walter, S.D., 1981, Personal and occupational factors associated with carpal tunnel syndrome. *J. Occup. Med.,* **23**(4), 225–258.

94. Armstrong, T.J. and Chaffin, D.B., 1979, Carpal tunnel syndrome and selected personal attributes. *J. Occup. Med.,* **21**(7), 481–486.

95. Ellis, M., 1951, Tenosynovitis of the wrist. *Br. Med. J.,* **2,** 777–779.

96. Barnes, C.G. and Currey, H.L.F., 1967, Carpal tunnel syndrome in rheumatoid arthritis, a clinical and electrodiagnostic survey. *Ann. Rheum. Dis.,* **26,** 226–233.

97. Sabour, M.S. and Fadel, H.H., 1970, The carpal tunnel syndrome—a new complication ascribed to the pill. *Am. J. Obstr. Gynecol.,* **107**(3), 1265–1267.

98. McGlothlin, J.D., Armstrong, T.J., Fine, L.J., Lifshitz, Y. and Silverstein, B., 1984, Can job changes initiated by a joint labor-management task force reduce the prevalence and incidence of cumulative trauma disorders of the upper extremity? *Proceedings of the 1984 International Conference on Occupational Ergonomics.* pp. 336–340.

Part II

Searching for Cumulative Trauma Indicators

Introduction

How do you determine whether the workers in a job, work group, plant, or company have symptoms of cumulative trauma? Similarly, how do you determine whether the workers are likely to develop CTDs in the near future?

The next three sections describe methods for collecting data that can help determine past or present occurrences of CTDs or help identify working conditions that may give rise to such disorders. These methods are briefly outlined as follows:

Reviewing available records

Existing medical and safety records are reviewed to identify past cases of CTDs. Often this information can be used to determine which current jobs pose a risk to workers.

Surveying the workers

Surveys are used to obtain information directly from the workers about the extent and location of their aches and pains. Workers can also provide detailed descriptions of their job activities and provide actual demonstrations of the motions used in their work. Survey information can be combined with the results of physical examinations of workers to assist in identifying current and past cases of CTDs.

Analyzing jobs

Each job or work task in which workers have experienced CTDs, or those jobs that may have a high-risk profile may be subjected to a systematic job analysis. A thorough analysis may include evaluation of the work methods, work stations and tools. The aim is to identify sources of biomechanical stress that may contribute to CTDs.

Each of these approaches has its advantages and disadvantages. Any thorough program of CTD evaluation and control usually involves components of all three surveillance techniques. A systematic approach for investigating the causes of CTDs often begins at the records review stage and progresses through the survey stage, and if warranted, is followed up with a specific job analysis. Such a progression is useful in establishing a more precise definition of the cumulative trauma problem and usually provides ample information for devising appropriate methods of control.

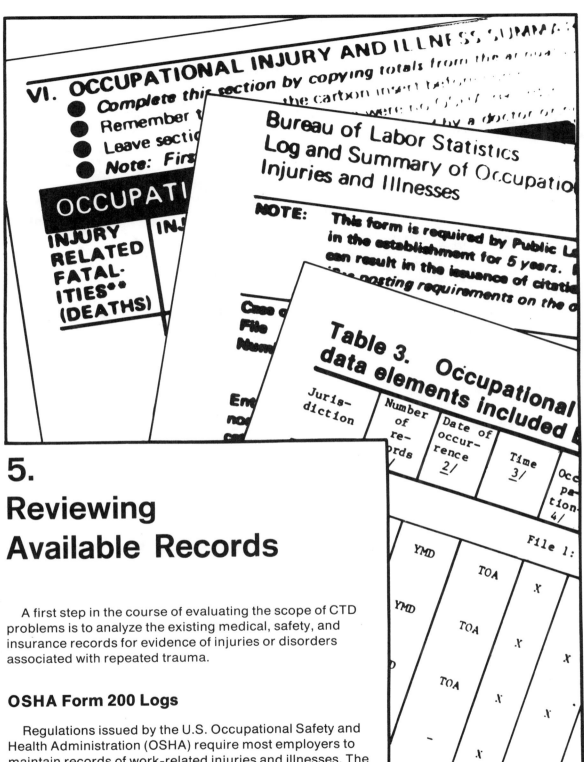

5.
Reviewing
Available Records

A first step in the course of evaluating the scope of CTD problems is to analyze the existing medical, safety, and insurance records for evidence of injuries or disorders associated with repeated trauma.

OSHA Form 200 Logs

Regulations issued by the U.S. Occupational Safety and Health Administration (OSHA) require most employers to maintain records of work-related injuries and illnesses. The standard form for keeping these records is OSHA No. 200, *Log and Summary of Occupational Injuries and Illnesses*. All on-the-job illnesses and injuries must be recorded on this form, which is shown in Table 2.

The instructions for completing Form 200 are somewhat ambiguous as to whether CTDs are occupational injuries or occupational illnesses. An occupational injury is defined as "any injury such as a cut, fracture, sprain, amputation, etc., which

Table 2.　Log and summary of occupational injuries and illnesses (OSHA Form 200).

Bureau of Labor Statistics
Log and Summary of Occupational
Injuries and Illnesses

U.S. D

Company Name		
Establishment Name		
Establishment Address		

NOTE:	This form is required by Public Law 91-596 and must be kept in the establishment for 5 years. Failure to maintain and post can result in the issuance of citations and assessment of penalties. *(See posting requirements on the other side of form.)*	RECORDABLE CASES: You are required to record information about every occupational death, every nonfatal occupational illness, and those nonfatal occupational injuries which involve one or more of the following loss of consciousness, restriction of work or motion, transfer to another job, or medical treatment (other than first aid) *(See definitions on the other side of form.)*

Case or File Number	Date of Injury or Onset of Illness	Employee's Name	Occupation	Department	Description of Injury or Illness	Extent of and Outcome	
						Fatalities	Nonfatal
Enter a nondupli-cating number which will facilitate com-perisons with supple-mentary records.	Enter Mo./day.	Enter first name or initial, middle initial, last name.	Enter regular job title, not activity employee was per-forming when injured or at onset of illness. In the absence of a formal title, enter a brief description of the employee's duties	Enter department in which the employee is regularly employed or a description of normal workplace to which employee is assigned, even though temporarily working in another depart-ment at the time of injury or illness	Enter a brief description of the injury or illness and indicate the part or parts of body affected.

Typical entries for this column might be Amputation of 1st joint right forefinger, Strain of lower back; Contact dermatitis on both hands, Electrocution—body | Injury Related

Enter DATE of death

Mo./day/yr | Injuries W

Enter a CHECK if injury involves days away from work, or days of restricted work activity, or both |
(A)	(B)	(C)	(D)	(E)	(F)	(1)	(2)
					PREVIOUS PAGE TOTALS　➡		
					TOTALS (Instructions on other side of form.)　➡		

OSHA No. 200

FOLD

Certification of Ann

OSHA No 200

results from a work accident or from an exposure in the workplace." An occupational illness is defined as "any abnormal condition or disorder, other than one resulting from an occupational injury, caused by exposure to environmental factors associated with employment." Several categories of occupational illnesses are listed, including "disorders associated with repeated motion, vibration, or pressure." These disorders are summarized and recorded on OSHA Form 200 under item

7f. The repeated trauma category, however, also includes hearing loss, so each case must be reviewed before it is counted.

The left side of the Form 200 (see Table 2) is particularly useful for identifying cases of CTDs. The right side of the form (not shown) is posted for the employees to review, which also serves as a summary of the injury and illness record for the company. The following procedure may be used to extract information from the form:

(1) Scan column F (Description of Injury or Illness) for all injuries or illnesses of the upper extremities *not* caused by accidents. Common diagnostic terms include: tendinitis, synovitis, arthritis, strain, etc., for the peripheral nervous system (e.g., numbness, tingling, nerve entrapments such as carpal tunnel syndrome, etc.). Note that cases are frequently misclassified, e.g., contusion instead of repeated trauma. Finally, some disorders will be vaguely defined as "persistent intermittent pain in the wrist and hand."

(2) If the information in column F indicates a case of upper extremity CTD, record the associated data in column D (Occupational Title) and column E (Department). These items may be very useful in identifying areas in a plant where CTDs are a serious problem.

(3) Finally, record the date of the injury or illness given in column B. This information may be useful in evaluating how changes in procedures and equipment affect the occurrence of CTDs.

The effectiveness of the OSHA Form No. 200 is limited by local practices of recording injuries and illnesses. Some plants record only those visits to the medical department that are clearly related to work activities. The logs kept at these plants could miss many CTD cases that were dismissed as due to off-the-job activities. Other plants record all visits to the medical department. The logs kept at these locations are more likely to reveal CTDs that are potentially occupational in origin.[1]

To ensure that complete logs are kept, plant medical personnel should be trained to recognize and record all visits that might be related to cumulative trauma problems. The person's work activity should also be recorded at the time of the visit, as well as any motions or postures that may affect the symptoms.

Plant medical records

If a company is large enough to have a clinic staffed by trained medical personnel, it may be possible to obtain information on CTDs by reviewing employee medical records. In many places, every visit to the company clinic is recorded in the employee's medical file and a monthly summary is available.[2] Typically, the information is similar to the entry data on the OSHA Form 200. It will include items such as the date of the visit, the occupational title at the time of the visit, the department or location where the patient worked, and a brief description of the injury or illness. Numeric codes may be used for recording injuries and illnesses such as the International Classification of Disease (ICD) system.[3]

The entry may also include a brief description of any treatment given, and any medications or work restrictions prescribed. In order to ensure the privacy rights of individuals, their medical records should be regarded as confidential information and secured accordingly.

These records vary from plant to plant in their usefulness. They may or may not include important information such as the reason for the visit to the clinic, the date, the job, or the department. The clinic staff may also lack the experience or training to identify CTDs or to determine whether the disorder is work-related. Again, these factors may influence the quality and utility of the existing medical records for assessing the extent of CTDs at a given worksite.

A problem in large plants with hundreds of employees is the sheer number of records that may have to be reviewed to uncover CTD cases. Unless the records have been entered into a computer file and can be accessed with data base software, the task of reviewing all records may be too time-consuming to be practical. An alternative is to use a random sampling technique to identify CTD cases.

Worker compensation records

Workers' compensation insurance records can be used to ascertain some of the costs resulting from CTDs. These costs may be broken down into two areas:

(1) Medical costs — Any payments made to outside hospitals, clinics, physicians, and other licensed medical personnel for the diagnosis and treatment (including surgery) of CTDs. If required, rehabilitation costs (such as occupational therapy) are included in this category.

(2) Disability costs — Any payments made directly to the injured worker for lost work time and payments made as a lump sum settlement for permanent disability.

The actual costs of a CTD are higher than those covered by workers' compensation insurance because insurance does not cover medical treatments rendered directly by the employer, and many employers supplement the disability coverage provided by the insurance carrier. Finally, workers' compensation statistics do not include the costs of cases that are not recognized as being occupationally caused. These cases are paid for directly by the injured worker or by comprehensive health insurance, which may be provided by the employer as a fringe benefit.

To determine workers' compensation costs associated with CTDs, records should be reviewed on a regular basis. Although considerable variability exists in the format of forms used in different states and by different insurance carriers, all forms will have an entry for a description of the illness or injury. This entry should be checked to see if the claim was filed for any disorder that might result from cumulative trauma (see Part I, Chapter 3 for a description of common CTDs). If so, the claim should be checked to make certain that the disorder did not result from an overt accident. If this requirement is satisfied, exposure information such as occupational title, department, etc., should be extracted from the claim.

Workers' compensation reports are quite useful in estimating some of the costs associated with CTDs and in identifying departments and job titles where these costs are high. On the other hand, workers' compensation reports describe only the most severe and advanced problems, and they may fail to identify problems which are in an early developmental stage.

Safety and accident reports

Accident reports and other records maintained by a plant's safety department are typically designed to record information associated with accidents. Because CTDs develop over an extended period of time and are caused by what are often considered normal activities, rather than mishaps, safety records are usually a poor source for documenting the extent of CTDs.

Payroll records

Payroll records are useful for obtaining information on the number of hours worked, but will seldom tell how much time is spent on each job. This computation serves as a crude measure of exposure potential and can be used to compare plants or jobs in terms of incidence rates of all forms of disorders, including those of cumulative trauma.

Payroll records may also be useful in identifying job titles or departments where there are high absentee or turnover rates. Although high turnover can result from several causes, physical stress is a common reason for leaving a job. Workers may choose to quit or bid out of those jobs that cause CTDs if less stressful jobs are available.

Minimum information required for evaluating records

To determine how many workers have symptoms or have been diagnosed as having a form of CTD, the following information is needed. Much of it is available from one or more of the sources described above:

(1) The total number of CTD cases reported.
(2) The date each case was reported.
(3) The department (or the specific job) of the injured worker.
(4) The number of workers on the same job or in the same department.

This information can be used to calculate the **incidence rate** or the number of CTDs per department or job for a specific time period. To compare various jobs or departments, the percentage of workers who had CTDs must be calculated.

First, some definitions are needed. The **incidence** of a disorder is **the number of new cases that come into being during a specified period of time**. The period of time is measured in calendar time (usually a year) and in exposure hours to a job. This calculation is usually done by estimating that each worker works 2000 hours per year (8 hours a day, 5 days a week, 50 weeks a year). Overtime would make the figure higher.

The formula for calculating incidence rates is as follows:

$$\text{Incidence rate} = \frac{\text{Number of new cases per year} \times 200{,}000 \text{ work hours}}{\text{Number of workers in dept} \times 2000 \text{ hours}}$$

(200,000 work hours is used to approximate 100 workers per year)

Example 1

Department X, with 907 workers, reported 21 cases of shoulder tendinitis in 1983. The department worked no overtime, so the figure of 2000 hours per worker is used. The incidence rate for shoulder tendinitis in 1983 would therefore be:

$$(21 \times 200{,}000) \text{ divided by } (907 \times 2000) = 2 \cdot 31$$
or 2·31 cases per 100 workers per year

Example 2

Department Y, with 29 workers, reported 2 cases of carpal tunnel syndrome in 1983. The incidence rate would therefore be:

$$(2 \times 200{,}000) \text{ divided by } (29 \times 2000) = 6 \cdot 89$$
or 6·89 cases per 100 workers per year

The number of workers in a department or plant can yield an approximation of total work hours, but the number of workers may fluctuate from month to month or from year to year. In addition, there may be either layoffs or overtime work. Often it is possible to obtain the **actual** number of hours worked by department and by the entire plant from the payroll or engineering departments. If the actual hours worked are used, the formula for calculating the incidence rates is:

$$\text{Incidence rate} = \frac{\text{Number of the new cases} \times 200{,}000 \text{ hours}}{\text{Total hours worked}}$$

Consider the information presented in Table 3 for Plant Z. The plant employed an average of 1450 workers during 1981 in three different departments. A review of the OSHA Form 200 records revealed that there were 36 new cases of tendinitis in the plant during the year. According to payroll records, a total of 2·9 million hours were worked. The table also gives the number of employees, tendinitis cases, and work hours for each of the three departments. The incidence rate is calculated for the whole plant and for each department using the above formula.

Table 3.   Annual tendinitis incidence rates in Plant Z

Item	Dept. A	Dept. B	Dept. C	Total Plant
Employees	450	300	700	1450
Hours worked	900,000	600,000	1,400,000	2,900,000
Tendinitis cases	22	4	10	36
Incidence rate per 100 workers/year	4·88	1·33	1·42	2·48

Table 3 shows that the rate of tendinitis cases in department A was more than three times the rate in departments B or C. Initial information such as this would be helpful in directing attention to department A for more in-depth study of the problems.

This type of procedure allows comparisons between and within the same departments from year to year. A plant-wide incidence rate is used as a baseline from which to evaluate specific departments or jobs. However, if the plant-wide rate itself is high, it may not be an acceptable comparison. **A plant-wide rate of 6 cases per 200,000 work hours has been used by some as an acceptable base line rate.** Other investigators consider this to be excessive.[4]

Conclusions

Although a thorough review of existing medical and production records is a necessary first step in any investigation of CTDs, it will seldom provide the type of conclusive information necessary to accurately assess the extent or potential for CTDs in the work force. A main problem is that CTDs are not always recognized as being work-related, and therefore many cases go unreported. Hence, plant or group statistics compiled for CTDs often fail to identify those jobs or workers who may be experiencing symptoms or who are future candidates for the disorders.

Any review of records should be done very carefully and interpreted with caution. In general, this process should be considered only a starting point for a subsequent worksite investigation and analysis. Furthermore, companies or unions who desire in-depth analyses of plant records for indications of CTDs should consult with specialists who have experience in surveillance research.

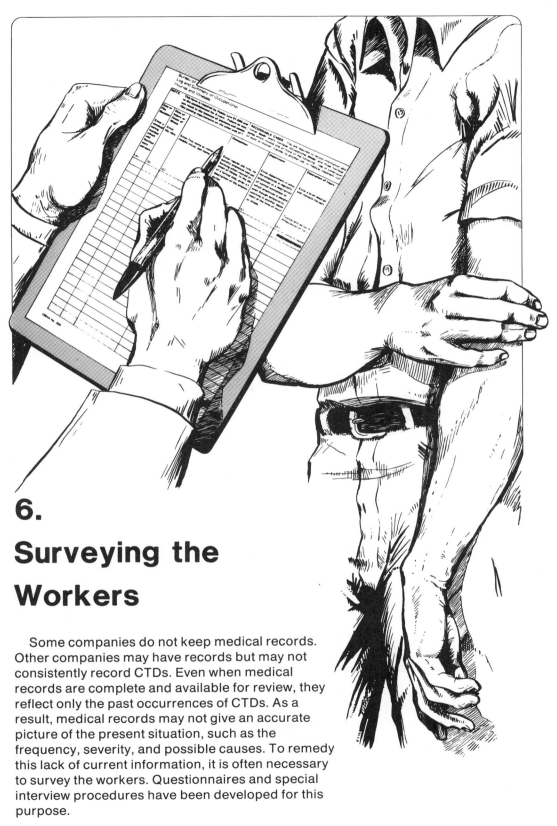

6.

Surveying the Workers

Some companies do not keep medical records. Other companies may have records but may not consistently record CTDs. Even when medical records are complete and available for review, they reflect only the past occurrences of CTDs. As a result, medical records may not give an accurate picture of the present situation, such as the frequency, severity, and possible causes. To remedy this lack of current information, it is often necessary to survey the workers. Questionnaires and special interview procedures have been developed for this purpose.

A main limitation of surveys and questionnaires is that they rely on the worker's recognition of, and willingness to report his or her health condition. Moreover, in the early stages of CTDs, many of the symptoms are transient and occur predominantly at night. Hence, the worker may not recall or recognize the significance of the symptoms during the day at the time of an interview or survey. In cases where more verifiable information is needed about existing and developing CTDs, a medical screening examination may need to be conducted.

Surveys and questionnaires

The survey can assist in identifying new or preclinical cases of CTDs in the workforce. Since almost all types of CTDs will produce some symptoms of pain or discomfort, the most direct approach is to ask workers if they experience pain or other symptoms in their upper extremities. Most pain surveys are usually sensitive to CTDs, but are poor at discriminating or diagnosing a specific disorder. Perhaps, the major strength of the survey approach is in collecting data on the **number of workers** that may be experiencing some form of CTD.

A survey is also a good method for identifying areas or jobs where potential CTD problems exist. For example, a high level of reported pain symptoms by various workers on a specific job would indicate the need for further investigation of that job including aspects of work place layout, equipment design, or work methods.

A typical questionnaire is shown below. These questions are designed to disclose the nature (pain, tingling, swelling, stiffness) and the location of symptoms. In addition, it is advisable to ask questions regarding systemic diseases or conditions. Questions are also needed to determine whether workers have ever been told by a physician that they had any of the following conditions: rheumatoid arthritis, hypertension, diabetes, thyroid disorders, lupus, gout or kidney disease. It may be necessary to inquire about oral contraceptive use or pregnancy among women experiencing symptoms of carpal tunnel syndrome. A number of these factors have been associated with CTD symptoms, but as yet, the role of any of these factors in the development of CTDs is unclear.

The results of a survey must be interpreted with caution. Tolerance of pain varies considerably from person to person and this will affect responses. Furthermore, since the survey is given to active workers, the reported symptoms are not disabling. A positive response only implies that the worker is experiencing noticeable discomfort.

Most survey instruments evolve over time as a consequence of trial and error. Surprisingly few people outside of the social and behavioral sciences are aware of the vast literature from the psychometric field on survey design and validation.[5] Examples of important factors that should be considered in designing surveys include: the reading level (or primary language) of those responding, the length of the questionnaire, the wording of the instructions given to the worker, and the time and method of administration (oral versus written). Fortunately, a number of reference sources are available that provide useful information on how to conduct surveys and administer various comfort rating scales.[6]

One survey method that requires a minimum of explanation is the use of a **body parts map** (Figure 11). The worker circles or

Sample questionnaire for cumulative trauma disorders

		No	Yes
(1)	Within the past month, have you had repeated feelings of numbness, tingling, or "pins and needles" sensations in one or both hands?	[ ]	[ ]
(2)	Within the past month, have you had repeated feelings of soreness or pain in either forearm or elbow?	[ ]	[ ]
(3)	Within the past month, have you had repeated feelings of pain discomfort, burning, or tingling in your shoulders?		
	Left	[ ]	[ ]
	Right	[ ]	[ ]
(4)	Have any of the above symptoms (numbness, tingling, soreness, or pain) caused you to be awakened while sleeping?	[ ]	[ ]
(5)	What time does your discomfort regularly occur?		
	Mornings	[ ]	[ ]
	Afternoons	[ ]	[ ]
	Evenings	[ ]	[ ]
	Night	[ ]	[ ]
(6)	Does discomfort in your wrist, arm, or shoulder interfere with your daily activities (eating, writing, sports, etc.)?	[ ]	[ ]
(7)	Have you ever received medical treatment for this pain and/or discomfort?	[ ]	[ ]
(8)	Have you ever received medical help (either company or private doctor) for any of the following:		
	Carpal tunnel syndrome?	[ ]	[ ]
	Ganglionic cysts?	[ ]	[ ]
	Tendinitis?	[ ]	[ ]
(9)	If yes to (8), have you ever had surgery for any of these conditions?	[ ]	[ ]
(10)	Does your present job require arm, hand, or finger actions to be repeated many times each hour and work shift?	[ ]	[ ]

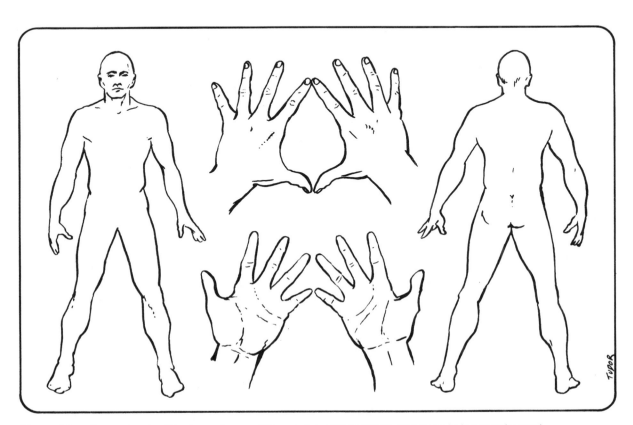

Figure 11. Example of a "Body-parts map" for workers' to indicate where pain is experienced.

places a mark on the part of the body where the pain or soreness is experienced. Depending on the type of work being evaluated and the need to delineate specific body regions, the body map can be divided into sections by drawing lines that separate various anatomical parts, such as the neck, shoulder, upper arm, lower arm, wrist, etc. By counting the incidence of any non-zero body part discomfort-reading for each body part and dividing by the number of times the map was administered, a simple measure of body part discomfort can be obtained. The notion is that sources of chronic discomfort or soft tissue soreness signal the existence of, or potential for, CTDs. Techniques for using and interpreting body part maps are described elsewhere.[7]

Medical screening exams

Medical screening examinations are particularly useful when the reported symptoms suggest that disorders are in the beginning stages and there are few documented cases of existing disorders. Based on the initial employee survey, trained medical personnel can examine people with a set of simple testing maneuvers to elicit a more accurate picture of the nature and severity of problems that may exist. For example, if an employee reports pain in the wrist, the following test, illustrated in Figures 12a and 12b, might be used.

(1) Passive wrist flexion and extension
(2) Passive ulnar and radial deviation
(3) Resisted flexion and extension
(4) Resisted ulnar and radial deviation
(5) Finklestein's test for De Quervain's disease[8]
(6) Phalen's test for carpal tunnel syndrome[9]

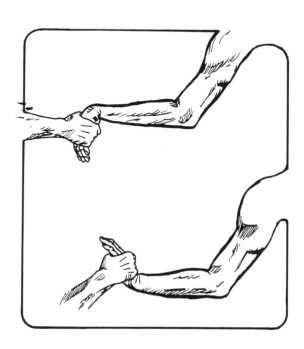

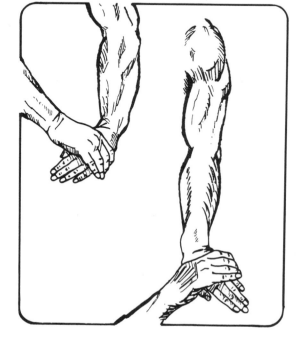

PASSIVE WRIST FLEXION AND EXTENSION   PASSIVE ULNAR AND RADIAL DEVIATION

Figure 12a.   Test motions for diagnosing wrist pain.

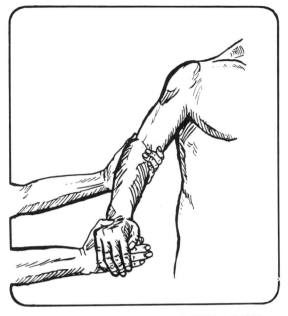

RESISTED FLEXION AND EXTENSION

Figure 12a.   continued.

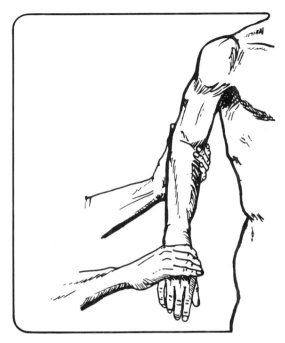

RESISTED ULNAR AND RADIAL DEVIATION

FINKLESTEIN'S TEST

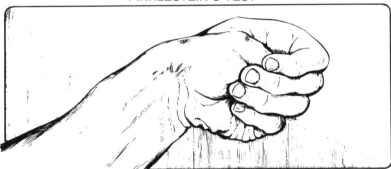

PHALEN'S TEST

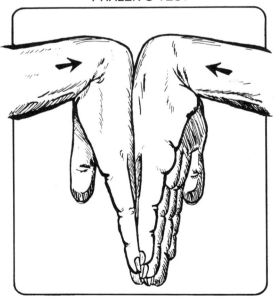

Figure 12b.   Test motions for diagnosing wrist pain.

Similarly, an evaluation of shoulder problems can be made for the most common disorders with the following motions:

(1) Touching the top of the head
(2) Scratching the back
(3) Forward flexion
(4) Resisted abduction
(5) Resisted supination

If the worker can perform these motions without limitation of movement or pain, no major problem is likely to be present. If there is pain or limitation, further evaluation by a physician is necessary. Appendix B provides a description of common diagnostic and treatment procedures for CTDs.

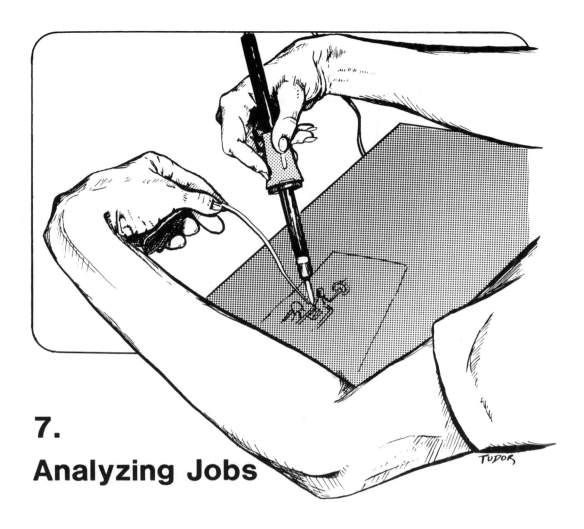

7.

Analyzing Jobs

Job analysis is useful for identifying sources of cumulative trauma before CTDs are manifested in claims.[10] Moreover, a job analysis can be used to evaluate improvements in job and tool redesign without having to wait until claims are actually reduced. Ideally, a job analysis should include a method for measuring the worker's exposure to each of the major biomechanical risk factors: force, posture, and repetition. The exposure should then be compared to known human capabilities to compute an injury probability. Since, however, there is limited dose-response data to establish a CTD risk, a series of similar jobs may have to be analyzed to determine what are acceptable postures or safe levels of force and frequency.[11] Hence, a job analysis is not only needed to identify the exposure to risk factors in problematic jobs, but is useful for documenting jobs that illustrate safe levels of task factors and effective work design.

A job analysis can be conducted in two ways. The first method is patterned after the traditional **work-methods analysis** and is particularly appropriate for new or unusually complex jobs. The second, and perhaps the most direct approach, is to use an ergonomic **checklist**. Examples of both methods are provided.

To perform a work-methods analysis a complete task description is needed to catalogue work content. This may include information derived from company production records, and video tapes of the job. Once the job components are documented, awkward postures, high repetition, and even excessive mechanical forces and stresses can be more readily identified. The most difficult task is to determine if those biomechanical risk factors pose demands that exceed acceptable ranges of human capacity, as limited by the design of the existing work station and tools. Fortunately, certain anthropometric and ergonomic guidelines are available to assist in that judgement. In the event that the existing guidelines are deficient, the profile of risk factors from suspect jobs can be compared with the profile from similar "safe" jobs where CTDs have not occurred.[12]

Work-Methods Analysis

The job is described as a set of tasks. Each task is defined in terms of a series of steps or elements.[13] Elements are described as fundamental movements or acts (reaching, grasping, moving, etc.) required to perform a job. A list of such work elements is shown in Table 4 as proposed by Gilbreth, a pioneer in the field of work analysis. The elements of Gilbreth's system are called Therbligs. Gilbreth's work served as the foundation for a widely used motion classification system called Methods–Time Measurement system (MTM). This system relies on a description of manual activities with reference to a defined set of elemental motions.[14] Elements are determined by observing the job or by observing videotapes of the job played in slow motion. The time required to complete one sequence of elements (the cycle time) is measured using a stop watch while actually observing the job, or by viewing videotapes played back in slow motion.

Tasks are defined as elements that are performed, usually in the same sequence. Examples of tasks might include getting a pallet, loading a pallet, cleaning a work area, stuffing a circuit board, sanding a part, etc. Tasks are determined from available

Table 4.   Gilbreth's table of work elements[13]

Element	Description
Search	Looking for something with the eyes or hand.
Select	Locating one object (that is) mixed with others.
Grasp	Touching or gripping an object with the hand.
Reach	Moving of the hand to some object or location.
Move	Movement of some object from one location to another.
Hold	Exerting force to hold an object on a fixed location.
Position	Moving an object in a desired orientation.
Inspect	Examining an object by sight, sound, touch, etc.
Assemble	Joining together two or more objects.
Disassemble	Separating two or more objects.
Use	Manipulating a tool or device with the hand.
Unavoidable delay	Interrupting work activity because of some factor beyond the worker's control.
Avoidable delay	Interrupting work activity because of some factor under the worker's control.
Plan	Performing mental process that precedes movement
Rest to overcome fatigue	Interrupting work activity to overcome the effects of repeated exertions or movements.

job descriptions, talking to supervisors and workers, and observing the job as it is performed. The time required to perform each task is best determined from available time-study or production records, but can also be estimated from direct observations with a stop watch.[15]

Examples of job analysis

To illustrate the work methods procedure, two examples are provided: bottle packing and sanding parts.

Bottle packing

The elements required to get a bottle from a moving conveyor and put it into a box (Figure 13 a) are as follows:

(1) **Reach** for bottles
(2) **Grasp** two bottles
(3) **Move** bottles to box
(4) **Position** bottles in box
(5) **Release** bottles

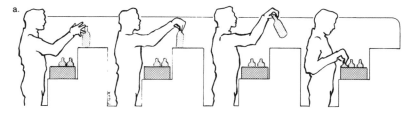

Figure 13a.   Elements required for bottle packing. Bottles are taken from a moving conveyor and placed in a carton.

Only one list of elements is required, since both hands do the same things; two lists are used when the right and left hands do different things, such as in the second example:

Sanding parts

The elements required to sand the edge of a fiber glass part (Figure 13 b) are as follows:

	Left hand	Right hand
(1)	**Reach** for part	**Hold** sander
(2)	**Grasp** part	**Hold** sander
(3)	**Move** part	**Hold** sander
(4)	**Position** part	**Hold** sander
(5)	**Hold** part	**Hold** sander to part
(6)	**Hold** part	**Move** sander over surface 5 times
(7)	**Move** to pallet	**Hold** sander
(8)	**Position** on pallet	**Hold** sander
(9)	**Release** part	**Hold** sander

Risk factor analysis

After elements of the job have been described and timed, the work content should be analyzed with respect to potential biomechanical risk factors for CTDs. A risk factor is defined as

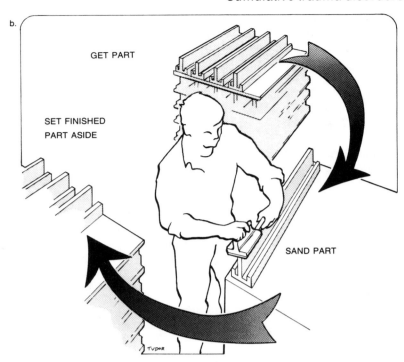

13b. Elements required for sanding a fiberglass part. Fiberglass parts are taken from one pallet, sanded on the bench, and stacked on another pallet.

an attribute or exposure that increases the probability of the disease or disorder.[17] Biomechanical risk factors for CTDs include repetitive and sustained exertions, awkward postures, and high mechanical forces. In addition, vibration, and low temperatures may accelerate the development of CTDs.

A brief descriptive phrase should be provided for each work element where biomechanical risk factors are evident. The analysis of the bottle packing example (Figure 13 a) revealed a number of awkward postures. They are:

> **Reach** — elbow above mid-torso height
> **Grasp** — elbow above mid-torso height pinching the bottles
> **Position** — inward rotation of forearm with flexed wrist; sharp edge on container rubs on base of palm.

Similarly, the potential risk factors identified in the sanding task, illustrated in Figure 13 b, are listed for each of three sub-tasks.

> **Grasp, Move,** and **Hold** part:
> —pinching part
> —stress concentrations from sharp edges of part
>
> **Hold** and **Move** sander:
> —pinching sander
> —sharp edges on sander handle
>
> **Move** sander:
> —sustained static effort to support sander, airline
> —inward rotation of forearm with wrist flexion
> —pinching sander
> —sharp edges on handle
> —vibration
> —cold exhaust air on fingers

Both of these examples illustrate the advantage of using work methods analysis to break complex motion patterns into manageable units. Potential biomechanical risk factors are usually apparent at this stage.

Checklist items for worksites

As an alternative or supplement to conducting work-methods analyses, checklists may be used to itemize undesirable worksite conditions or worker activities that contribute to injury. Examples of checklists can be found in a number of reference texts on human factors and ergonomics.[18,19,20] If the goal is to identify risk factors for CTDs, then the checklist should be customized to include a list of the biomechanical risk factors. For each risk factor, specific job attributes should also be included to focus the effort. For example, the risk factor of force is relevant to holding, assembling and pinching. Similarly, posture problems are associated with reaching, inspecting and assembling.

Although most checklists are problem oriented, they may also restrict observations of situations not specifically described. The best solution is to customize existing checklists to meet the specific needs of different worksites or departments. A checklist for an office will emphasize different job attributes and risk factors than one for manufacturing. Before using a checklist at a new job site, a walk through survey should be conducted to determine if the checklist encompasses items that identify the needed mix of risk factors and job attributes. Most ergonomic checklists will have items that cover the following four problematic work conditions:

(1) *Crowding or cramping of the worker*.
Work area layout that may force the worker to stoop or bend to fit the workspace or to unnecessarily constrain movements.
(2) *Twisting or turning*.
Placement of tools and materials that may force the worker to twist the spine to see and reach what is needed for the job.
(3) *Repeated reaching motions*.
Work area layout that may force the worker to stretch and lean to reach and grasp needed objects or controls.
(4) *Misalignment of body parts*.
Arrangement of the work area that causes the worker to frequently have one shoulder higher than the other, or have the spine or neck bent to one side or the other.

An example of a "yes–no" checklist useful for walk through surveys is shown in Table 5. With a two-choice checklist a quantitative score can be readily derived for each risk factor and each job. The final score is the percentage of the items scored as "yes". For the checklist in Table 5 a score of 100% suggests minimal risk for CTDs.

The following section provides a brief review of some of the rationale and procedures for evaluating work which poses a risk for CTDs. Following the theme of this manual, biomechanical risk factors are examined with respect to stressful postures, excessive force and high repetition or frequency.

Table 5.   Michigan's checklist for upper extremity cumulative trauma disorders*

Risk factors	No	Yes
1. Physical stress		
1.1 Can the job be done without hand/wrist contact with sharp edges?	[ ]	[ ]
1.2 Is the tool operating without vibration?	[ ]	[ ]
1.3 Are the worker's hands exposed to temperature >21 °C (70 °F)	[ ]	[ ]
1.4 Can the job be done without using gloves?	[ ]	[ ]
2. Force		
2.1 Does the job require exerting less than 4·5 Kg (10 lbs) of force?	[ ]	[ ]
2.2 Can the job be done without using finger pinch grip?	[ ]	[ ]
3. Posture		
3.1 Can the job be done without flexion or extension of the wrist?	[ ]	[ ]
3.2 Can the tool be used without flexion or extension of the wrist?	[ ]	[ ]
3.3 Can the job be done without deviating the wrist from side to side?	[ ]	[ ]
3.4 Can the tool be used without deviating the wrist from side to side?	[ ]	[ ]
3.5 Can the worker be seated while performing the job?	[ ]	[ ]
3.6 Can the job be done without "clothes wringing" motion?	[ ]	[ ]
4. Workstation hardware		
4.1 Can the orientation of the work surface be adjusted?	[ ]	[ ]
4.2 Can the height of the work surface be adjusted	[ ]	[ ]
4.3 Can the location of the tool be adjusted?	[ ]	[ ]
5. Repetitiveness		
5.1 Is the cycle time longer than 30 seconds?	[ ]	[ ]
6. Tool design		
6.1 Are the thumb and finger slightly overlapped in a closed grip?	[ ]	[ ]
6.2 Is the span of the tool's handle between 5 and 7 cm (2–2¾ inches)?	[ ]	[ ]
6.3 Is the handle of the tool made from material other than metal?	[ ]	[ ]
6.4 Is the weight of the tool below 4 kg (9 lbs)**	[ ]	[ ]
6.5 Is the tool suspended?	[ ]	[ ]

["No" responses are indicative of conditions associated with the risk of CTDs.]
   *Lifshitz, Y. and Armstrong, T., 1986, A design checklist for control and prediction of cumulative trauma disorders in hand intensive manual jobs, *Proceedings of the 30th Annual Meeting of Human Factors Society*, 837–841.
   **Note exceptions to the rule; see p. 108, first paragraph.

Evaluating stressful postures

Each major joint in the body has a wide range of movement. But any movement that over-extends a joint, that is, forces the joint beyond its natural range, can be harmful because some of the fibers that make up the tendons and ligaments may be over-stretched from chronic use and possibly torn.[21]

Since posture is an important consideration in the design of work procedures and equipment, portable videotape cameras are often used at the worksite to record the movements and postures of the worker's arms and hands during a series of job cycles. Later, the recorded work activity can be analyzed to determine the speed, angle and frequency of worker movement.[22]

The shoulder

Jobs that require the worker to habitually reach and work with the arms above the shoulder level (such as reaching up to remove or put parts on an overhead conveyor) are not only fatiguing, but have been associated with a range of disorders such as shoulder tendinitis or thoracic outlet syndrome.[23] Shoulder ailments can also be caused by repeated reaching behind the body or throwing parts over the shoulder into a bin behind the body. For example, the motion of sorting and moving merchandise past optical price-scanning screens may be responsible for some of the musculoskeletal problems experienced by cashiers in supermarkets (Figure 14).[24]

The elbow

Motions that are particularly stressful to the elbow include inward or outward rotation of the forearm when the wrist is bent. This movement stresses the tendons in the arm, leading to so-called tennis elbow or golfer's elbow.[25] Repetitive work that requires the elbow to be held straight and the arm extended is also likely to cause shoulder problems.

The muscles located in the forearm provide the major power and strength for the hand. They, like other muscles, are at their best mechanical advantage when in the midpoint of their normal range of movement, i.e., less tension is developed at lengths less than and greater than the resting length of the muscle. For example, when the arm is extended, the flexors of the forearm are at a mechanical disadvantage and can produce only weak lifting and pulling actions. A task requiring forceful lifting (or even using a screwdriver in this position) may overload the muscles and strain the arm.

The hand and wrist

The hand and wrist postures used by a worker on the job strongly influence the ability to reach, hold, and use equipment.

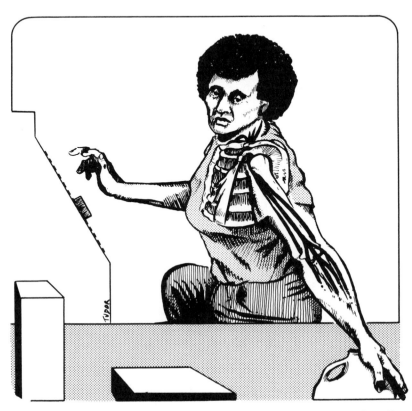

Figure 14. Arm position assumed by cashiers moving merchandise past an optical universal product coder (UPC).

Ultimately, these postures determine how long a worker can perform a job without adverse health effects such as fatigue and CTD.

Various tasks and tools frequently force the wrist to assume awkward postures. Wrist position is important because it affects the length–tension relationship of contracting muscles. As the angle of the joint increases or decreases beyond its midpoint (neutral position), there is a proportional decrease in effective strength. This means that more exertion or tendon tension is required to do a task with a bent wrist than is required to do the same task with a wrist in the neutral position. A number of wrist and finger postures have been identified as particularly stressful. They are listed below and illustrated in Figure 15.

Ulnar deviation — bending the wrist toward the little finger.
Radial deviation — bending the wrist toward the thumb.
Extension — bending the wrist up and back.
Flexion — bending the wrist down towards the palm.
Pinching — flexor surface of thumb is opposed to index finger.

A job, for example, that requires repeated ulnar deviation combined with supination (turning the palm up) often leads to tenosynovitis of the tendons on the back of the hand.[26] Examples would be looping wire with standard needle-nose pliers, inserting and starting screws by hand or rotating controls.

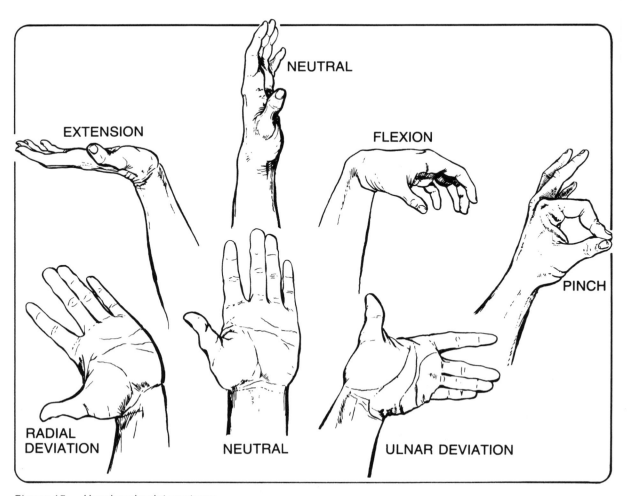

Figure 15.   Hand and wrist postures.

Strong radial deviation combined with pronation (palm down) can cause tennis elbow. Work strain or pain can often be felt in areas removed from the actual stress. In some cases, the wrist may be stressed, but it is the elbow that gets sore. Many common jobs require wrist radial deviation with pronation, for example, using a power sander or wire brush.[27]

Figure 16 a illustrates a common wrist posture adopted by workers boning turkey carcasses in a poultry processing plant. The combination of repetitive cutting motions and the need to forcefully bend the wrist to set the knife angle for cutting irritates the flexor tendons in the carpal tunnel of the wrist; a critical factor in causing tendinitis and carpal tunnel syndrome.[28] Figure 16 b shows a knife with a pistol grip that can also be used for cutting in the vertical plane that reduces the tendency to bend the wrist while cutting.

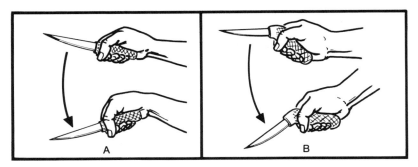

Figure 16(A).   Ulnar wrist deviation required to hold knife for boning turkey thighs;
(B)   Wrist posture can be controlled by changing shape of handle.

Finger and hand grasps

There are two basic types of grasps or ways of gripping an object: The **power grasp and the precision grasp**.[29] Examples of different grips are shown in Figure 17. The medial grasp is a power grasp, as in gripping a hammer. The pinch grasp (pulp and lateral) is useful for precise manipulations. Picking up a flat object from the table would be an example of the latter. A lateral or instrument grasp is classified as a precision grip. An example would be holding a piece of chalk or a key. Spherical or cylindrical grasps are sometimes considered power grasps, depending on the shape of the item to be grasped. An example would be turning a door handle to open a door.

In the power grasp, the thumb aligns the hand with the long axis of the forearm, and the wrist assumes a slight ulnar deviation. This posture may be harmful when combined with high movement frequency and the use of excessive force. Repetitive use of the pinch grasp also creates friction on the two tendons that control the thumb. Because the thumb tendons share a common sheath, tension levels are elevated by the two stretched tendons needed to maintain the pinch grip. The tendons will be further stressed if the task calls for pinching in combination with wrist flexion.

The grasping power of the hand is greatest when the hand is in the neutral position or slightly bent upwards (extended) and is

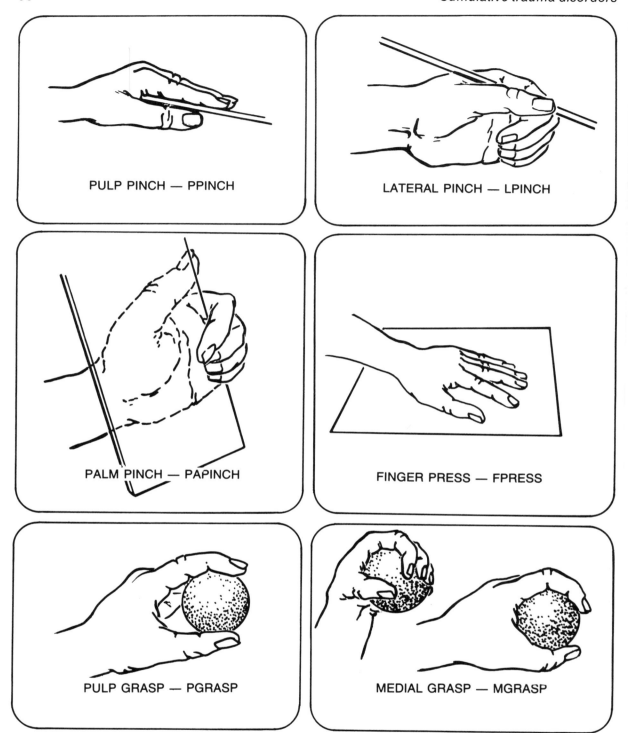

Figure 17.   Terminology for classifying various finger-closing postures.

reduced when the wrist is bent downward or from side to side.[30] Ulnar deviation may result in a loss of up to 25% of grip strength, and radial deviation may be associated with a loss of up to 20% of strength. Figure 18 illustrates the reduction in grip strength for various wrist postures as a percentage of the maximum grip force.[31]

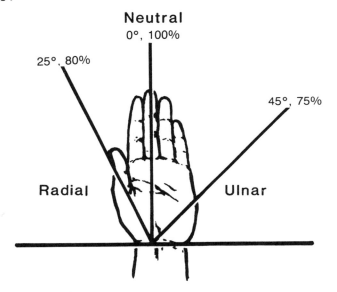

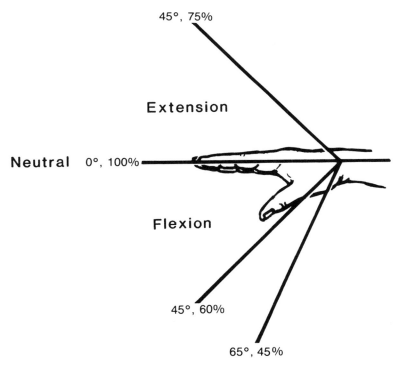

Figure 18.   Grip strength as a function of the degree of wrist deviation expressed as a percentage of power grip as measured in the neutral position.

Evaluating forces and muscle strengths

Unlike posture, which is relatively visible to an observer or can be recorded on video tape, the analysis of job forces or task loads is both more obscure and technically difficult. Furthermore, once force levels have been determined, the aversive impact of the force levels is dependent on the available muscle strength of the worker and how the task is performed.

Factors affecting force

The amount of force required to do a job depends, in part, on the properties of the tool or object manipulated: size and shape, effective weight, surface frictional characteristics and inertial effects. The effective weight is a function of the mass of the object and any moments or torque created during handling. A moment is created whenever an object is grasped and lifted away from its center of gravity. Inertia is a determining factor when the object is accelerating or decelerating.

Certain principles of mechanics must also be appreciated when the force requirements of a manual task are considered.[32] For example, the amount of force required to hold an object with the fingers is proportional to the force causing it to slip out of the hand, and inversely proportional to its slipperiness, or coefficient of friction (CF). The CF for a moist hand is about 2·0, whereas for a dry hand it is about 0·5. Hence, a dry hand is in fact more slippery than a moist hand. The fact that more force is required to grasp something with a dry hand than a moist hand is demonstrated by the ease in which a moistened finger can be used to turn the pages in a book as compared to a dry (slippery) finger.[33] Force can be reduced by using rubber covers, gloves, or handles. Slipperiness can be reduced by removing oil and grease from handles and hands.

The force causing an object to slip out of the hand can be estimated from its weight, the tightness of a fit or the power setting of a tool. Weight is related to the mass and number of objects held in the hand. Friction is related to the material properties of the handle and to the moistness of the skin. Forces can often be estimated from information about the task, such as the size and weight of a part or a tool. More strength is also required to lift a handful of parts than an individual part. In other cases, the force exerted with the hand is less obvious. Examples include buffing and grinding, sewing, and assembling parts.

Measuring force requirements

As noted, it is difficult to measure the force requirements of most jobs and also to determine the proportion of the worker's strength demanded to perform the job. Specialized procedures and modern electronic equipment are usually needed to obtain meaningful data. One such technique that has been extensively used in laboratory studies of muscle activity is **electromyography** (EMG). EMG works in much the same way that an electrocardiogram registers heart activity. Small metal disks are placed over the muscle groups. The electrical impulses given off by muscles during contraction are sensed and recorded by the EMG equipment for later analysis. By recording and comparing the activity of different muscle groups, a trained person can often determine which motions or body postures are overloading different muscles.[34]

Force and posture relationship

Certain work postures are more efficient than others, and consequently allow the same work to be done with less force exerted, or conversely require a smaller percentage of the worker's strength capacity. This is illustrated in Figure 19. On the

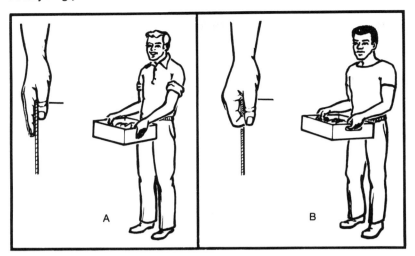

Figure 19. Two alternate hand postures or grips for holding: (A) pinch and (B) hook. The pinch grip requires more muscle strength, which stresses hand tendons and is more fatiguing than a hook grip.

left side of the figure, a worker is holding a box using a pinch grip. The absence of handles increases the load on the smaller finger and thumb flexors. On the right side of the figure, handles in the form of cutouts are provided allowing the worker to use a hook or power grip that effectively transfers the required force from the hands and forearms to the larger shoulder muscles. Studies show that the power grip provides a worker with more than five times the gripping strength of a precision grip.[35,36] Hence, the strength requirements of a task can be reduced, and the tendon loads lessened, if a task is performed using a larger muscle mass than a smaller one.

The relationship between force and the effect of body posture is also illustrated by a task that requires a worker to rotate his forearm in an outward direction. This motion relies predominantly on the biceps for its strength. By comparison, inward rotation of the forearm uses weaker muscles that fatigue more quickly. For example, using a screwdriver with the arm extended will cause the arm to fatigue sooner in the extended position than in the partially flexed position. A main reason is that the muscles in the forearm are weaker than the biceps.[37]

Evaluating frequency of movements

Repetitiveness can be defined biomechanically as the number of movements that occur in a given amount of time, or simply the time needed to complete the task, called the cycle time. A long cycle does not mean that the job is not repetitive, but that a sequence of steps is repeated to complete the overall cycle. This is illustrated in the bottle packing example, described above. Bottle packing requires 36 seconds to pack each case. Since, each case has 24 bottles, the "fundamental" cycle time is 1·5 seconds (36 divided by 24). A fundamental cycle is a work cycle that has a sequence of steps or elements (Therbligs) that repeat themselves within the cycle.

Similarly, with the example of sanding parts, 45 seconds are required to finish each part, but 30 of the 45 seconds are needed to move the sander 5 times. Hence, the fundamental cycle is closer to 6 seconds (30 divided by 5). These examples illustrate the importance of conducting a job analysis to evaluate the frequency of movements.

Most observers would judge the above examples as highly repetitive. There are, however, no guidelines or criteria for defining a task as either highly repetitive, or low in repetition. Faced with this problem, one investigative team developed a categorization procedure in which jobs were rated as either "high" or "low" in repetitiveness on the basis of estimated cycle time and the percentage of cycle time performing the same fundamental cycle. Cycle times of experienced operators were either measured by direct observation or from videotapes of the jobs. Information on work standards and production records were also used in obtaining estimates of cycle times.[38,39]

Jobs were classified as **low repetitive** if the cycle time was more than 30 seconds, or if less than 50% of the cycle time involved performing the same kind of fundamental cycle.

Jobs were classified as **high repetitive** if the cycle time was less than 30 seconds, or if more than 50% of the cycle time involved performing the same kind of fundamental cycle.

The findings from an independent assessment of the incidence of CTDs at the same plants indicated that workers in jobs that had been classified as high in repetition and force had a 31% greater risk for tendinitis than workers who had jobs classified as low in repetition and force levels.

In addition to repetition rate, the intensity and pace at which the worker is expected to work to meet production standards also has a significant effect on the development of CTDs. Recent studies indicate that some time standards may allow or even encourage workers to over-stress their body in pursuit of quotas. Working through breaks to achieve a quota is a common example.[40]

Evaluating physical fatigue

Fatigue is a complex problem that involves physiological and psychological effects. Physiological fatigue, or local fatigue, refers to excessive use of a muscle or body system. It may be experienced as a cramp in the small muscles of the hands which accompanies overuse of the fingers. There may also be more general fatigue encompassing loss of interest, diminished alertness, reduced perceptual capacity and faulty judgment. At the worksite general fatigue can lead to reduced performance, increased error rates and potential for mishaps.

Local fatigue may be further categorized as acute or chronic. The main distinction is that acute fatigue is relieved by rest, whereas chronic fatigue sets in when the recovery period between work sessions is insufficient to allow physiological adaptation. When local fatigue sets in, and muscles are not allowed to recover, muscles give up their share of the workload, and place **undue stress** on the other components, such as the ligaments. When ligaments are asked to do the work of muscles, they strain and tear more easily. Hence, chronic muscle fatigue may be viewed as a risk factor for CTDs.

In the simplest case, fatigue depends on how **hard** as well as how **long** a person works. For hand grip contractions, the intensity of a contraction is more critical in producing fatigue than the duration of the hand grip contraction by a factor of ten. In other words, the duration of work can be increased ten-fold and effort or fatigue will only increase five-fold, whereas by increasing the force ten-fold, effort or fatigue will increase fifty-fold. This suggests that in evaluating fatigue, at least for static tasks, load and duration are not interchangeable factors. The implication for work design is that fatigue may be reduced by reducing the load, while increasing the duration of work.[41]

There is a large body of literature on local muscle fatigue and its relationship to various static postures and repetitive motions.[42] Most of these studies clearly document those postures and force levels that produce high levels of local muscle effort. The inference is that excessive effort poses a strain to the musculoskeletal system that, over time, will translate into CTDs. Though this is a difficult association to establish in a direct manner, a number of worksite studies have been conducted that lend indirect support to this relationship.[43,44]

The rate of fatigue onset is also related to the intensity of work. Work intensity is often measured in terms of a percentage of maximum strength. The general finding is that most exertions below 15% of maximum strength will not be sustained long enough or frequently enough to produce objectionable fatigue. Studies have been conducted on repetitive exertions of given durations and intensity and with rest periods for single muscle groups.[45] Unfortunately, there are major difficulties associated with generalizing such results to specific work situations.

As a rule, objectionable discomfort is reached before the point of exhaustion. Therefore, endurance or fatigue curves are not very meaningful. Rather, time-to-discomfort curves are more realistic in determining work endurance.[46] In summary, most job evaluations calling for determinations of rest allowances will require actual on site measurements of the specific job demands as well as the assessment of worker discomfort levels.[47,48]

Evaluating work stations and worker posture

A thorough job analysis must also include a study of the work environment. A main feature of the work environment is the work station. This term denotes the workspace within the direct reach of the individual and includes all relevant work fixtures, such as the work table, stools or chairs as well as any supply and output containers.[49] Tools are not included.

Recent investigations of musculoskeletal complaints and poor performance indicate that a significant proportion of these problems can be traced to the faulty layout and design of work stations.[50,51,52] [Some solutions will be addressed in Part III: Preventing cumulative trauma disorders.]

Static Work

Discomfort and fatigue often arise from having to hold tensed muscles in a fixed or awkward position for long periods.

Examples of static work include holding the extended arms either forwards or sideways, and bending the head and neck forwards or backwards. Work conditions that are recognized as requiring considerable static hand-and-arm effort are defined as follows:[53]

(1) High effort lasting 10 seconds or more, e.g. holding an object of 4 kg.
(2) Moderate effort lasting 1 minute or more, e.g. holding an object of 2 kg.
(3) Slight effort lasting 4 minutes or more (about $\frac{1}{3}$ of maximum force).

Work postures involving elevated arms, such as the workers illustrated in Figure 20, may accelerate tendon degeneration by increasing the friction on the tendons. It may also cause muscle fatigue from the static-muscle effort needed to hold the arms overhead, which reduces the blood flow to the large muscles in the shoulder girdle: the trapezius, biceps brachii and deltoid. It is thought that the restricted blood flow is responsible, in part, for

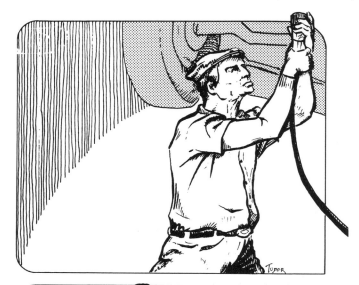

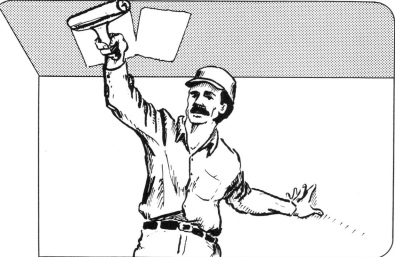

Figure 20.   Examples of overhead static-work that may cause nerves and adjacent blood vessels to be compressed between the neck and shoulder.

the familiar sensation of muscle burning — an indicator or warning sign to rest.

Muscles subjected to static work require more than 12 times longer than the original contraction-duration for complete recovery from fatigue.[54,55] Moreover, the muscles of the upper extremity cannot maintain a contraction level in excess of 20% of their strength for more than a few seconds without significant fatigue. Hence, in the absence of sufficient recovery time, prolonged and excessive static work will weaken joints, ligaments and tendons.[56]

The actual duration of exertion is dependent on the load and the individual muscle group. In general, the maximum holding time of a muscle group is related logarithmically to the proportion of maximum force that it is required to maintain. This is another way of saying that arithmetic increments in force are accompanied by geometric declines in holding time.[57]

Static work postures have been associated with the occurrence of degenerative tendinitis, tenosynovitis, insertion injuries and muscle induration.[58] Work that is repetitive or dynamic, by contrast, allows muscles to rhythmically contract and relax during work. Muscles involved in dynamic work are more resistant to fatigue and subsequent injury.

Work space and reaching distances

One of the major factors to consider in designing or evaluating a work space is the worker's physical dimensions. Most work stations are not adjustable to fit the wide range of differences in the height and weight of people who may be using them.[59] Work spaces are often designed for the mythical average person, which can be limiting to a large portion of the population. If a door, for example, was designed for the average person, 50% of the population would have to duck their heads when passing through.

In designing a work station, the goal should be to establish reach limits allowing objects to be grasped without excessive body motion or energy expenditure. This is particularly important when the worker is constrained to one seat location. A number of jobs require a seated worker to extend the arms forward, or bend the back forward or sideways to reach equipment or to lift parts. These jobs can be designed with optimal reach limits to avoid overextension or too much back bending and twisting.

Existing and proposed work stations should be evaluated for adequacy of anthropometric fit **during a normal work cycle**. The emphasis should be on obtaining functional measurements in contrast to static anthropometric measurements. Static measurements provide some information about the boundaries of the reach envelope, but they do not provide a basis for judging the types of work activities that can be safely and efficiently carried out at given distances from the body.

Reach limits can be determined either empirically through direct measurement of body parts, or estimated from existing anthropometric data tables of average body-link lengths.[60,61] In past years drawing-board manikins were used in conjunction with standard drafting techniques to estimate optimal work locations. Recently the manikin technique has been adapted to microcomputers and implemented with computer-aid drafting systems (CAD). CAD systems are more efficient because a variety of workstations and postures can be created without having to manually draw each configuration.[62]

Height of the work surface

The height of the work surface has a major impact on job performance and musculoskeletal problems. If the work surface is too high, the arms must be held away from the body (abducted) and the shoulders lifted. This can cause painful cramps in the shoulders and neck. If the work surface is too low, the worker must bend over, which can cause pain in the neck and lower back. Ideal surface height is a function of both the elbow height of the worker and the type of work.[63] Elbow height is determined with the elbows held close to the body and bent at 90 degrees (Figure 21). Factors that influence the type of work include: size of the work piece, the level of required manual effort, shape, weight and the type of motions required to accomplish the task. Some guidelines for establishing work height are provided in Part III.

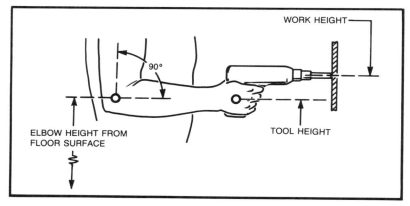

Figure 21. *Graphic aid for determining correct height, based on tool size.*

Sitting versus standing

Today the majority of workers are seated. The increase in clerical and information processing jobs relative to manufacturing jobs is responsible in part for this. Sitting is generally less fatiguing than standing, since only the weight of the upper torso must be supported. Of course, any sustained posture over time will eventually become fatiguing. For example, sitting in a poorly designed chair or in an unsupported sitting position can be extremely uncomfortable and encourages poor posture. This may lead to low back pain. Hence, whether a worker sits or stands, certain muscles will be fatigued.

A seated worker generally has greater stability and is able to perform jobs requiring precision or fine, manipulative movement, especially if provided with arm rests. If seating and other support is not provided, performance may suffer because more energy is required to maintain a standing posture. A special standing chair or stool offers another alternative for providing postural support.

Some tasks specifically call for the worker to stand so that he or she will be able to exert greater forces and move around more. The standing worker also has a greater area within his or her reach, which means that a larger work area can be covered than by the seated worker. As long as a person is standing, an outlay of static muscular effort is required to keep the joints of the feet, knees and hips in a fixed position. Thus, muscular stress is increased. A worker who stands also has a smaller area on which to support his or her body weight, namely, the feet, as compared to the area available to one who sits, the buttocks. Because of the smaller area of support, the standing worker has less margin-of-error to maintain balance. If standing is required, it should be alternated with sitting whenever possible. This will reduce fatigue by alternating the muscles used to maintain posture.[64]

Evaluating tools, handles and controls

The handle on a tool, a container or a machine control should be designed to fit the capabilities of the human hand and arm. In the past, craftsmen made or purchased their own tools. Since their tools represented a significant investment in the job, it was important that each tool be the right size, shape, and weight for the task. Finding the right tool, however, was often a matter of trial and error.

Today in a typical work place, tools are specified by an engineer, ordered by the procurement department, and handed out by a tool room attendant — none of whom uses them. It should come as no surprise then, that many tools do not fit the workers who use them.

Tools that are poorly designed for the worker and job may have a number of undesirable characteristics, including an awkward grip, a handle that causes the wrist to bend, a trigger requiring heavy pressure, a lack of balance, and low-frequency vibration.[65] For example, frequent and sustained contact with the hard, sharp edges of a hand-held tool, such as a pliers, may pinch the skin and tendon if sufficient strength is applied. This is illustrated in Figure 22a, and Insert b. The compression effect is significantly reduced, however, when the tool edge is rounded and smooth (Insert c, Figure 22). Hence, poorly designed tools may cause inflamed wrist tendons, obstruct the flow of blood in the palm, and cause fatigue from undernourished muscles. When compounded for months or years these conditions often lead to CTDs.[66,67]

Indicators of faulty tool selection or usage

A careful examination of body postures and accompanying work conditions may reveal that a faulty tool or control is being used. Examples of such conditions include:

(1) Static loading of arm and shoulder muscles.
(2) Awkward hand position, especially wrist deviation.
(3) Excessive or continuous pressure on the palm and fingers.

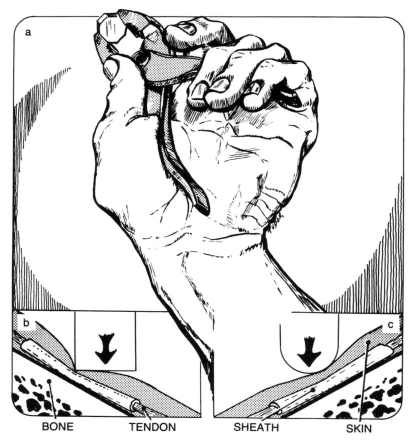

BONE   TENDON   SHEATH   SKIN

*Figure 22.   Example of how a hand tool can compress finger tendons
(a). A sharp-edged tool (b) is more likely to produce injury than a
rounded tool (c).*

(4) Exposure to vibration and cold from power tools.
(5) Pinch points with double-handled tools.
(6) Handles that require stretching of the hand to grip or high
     force to hold.

The routine use of improper tools can produce nearly the
same combination of stressful work patterns as faulty work
stations or work methods. Stressful work patterns that involve
the use of tools and controls include problems associated with
(1) arm and wrist orientation, (2) frequency of movement, and (3)
forces required by the task. Examples and a discussion of these
problems follow.

Tool-induced postures

One of the most common complaints about tools relates to the
location of the handle, which forces the worker to bend the wrist
when using the tool. If the tool is used repetitively with a bent
wrist, the tendons in the hand are strained and an inflammatory
condition is induced that can cause significant hand pain.[68]
Figure 23 illustrates a stressful **ulnar deviation** of the wrist. Such
postures are often assumed as a result of using the wrong-
shaped tool or handle while performing a task on a surface that
is either too high or too low.

The type of grip (precision or power) used on a tool also
determines to a large extent the angle of the wrist and elbow.

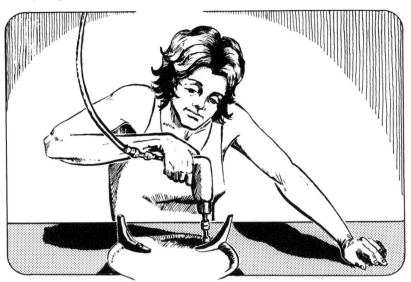

Figure 23. Stressful ulnar deviation associated with faulty tool and workstation layout.

When the wrist is fully extended, but not over-extended, grasping power is 100%, pinching or holding power is 50%, and manipulative effectiveness is 50%. When the wrist is fully flexed, the hand is close to 100% effective in manipulation, but has almost no holding power, i.e., grip strength is about half of what it is when in a neutral position.

Tools that cause ulnar deviation and/or palmar flexion, especially while rotating, may inflame wrist tendons and cause tenosynovitis. Inserting screws in holes, looping wire with pliers, and manipulating rotating controls are examples of this action. Tools that call for ulnar deviation coupled with supination (turning the palm up) of the wrist may also increase the risk of tenosynovitis. Tools that cause **radial deviation**, especially in combination with pronation and extension (rotating the wrist down), can lead to epicondylitis (tennis elbow). A main reason is that pressure is increased between the head of the radius and the capitulum of the humerus in the elbow.[69] This posture irritates the tendinous attachment of the finger extensor muscle on the outside of the elbow. Examples of tasks where tools may be used in this manner include: tightening or twisting covers, inserting components on a suspended assembly line, or cutting meat. In general, any tool that forces the wrist into an awkward posture will not only impede the transmission of the contractile force of the extensor/flexor muscles that control the hands, but is also likely to compress or irritate the median nerve or synovial tissues of the hand and arm.

Tool-related repetitive action

Repetitive finger action such as that required to operate triggers on tools may lead to a condition of "trigger finger" (a form of stenosing tenosynovitis crepitans). This condition is associated with the use of tools with handles too large for the worker's hand. This causes the worker to keep the end segments of the fingers flexed while the middle segment is kept straight in order to reach the trigger. A condition of chronic-flexor tension is induced, which, when combined with the repetitive finger flexing, irritates the tendon sheaths causing constriction of tendon action. As the tendon passes the site of obstruction, a click or snap is often produced.

Vibration has also been implicated in CTDs, although there is yet no conclusive evidence. Studies of forestry workers, however, suggest tool vibration may accelerate the onset of CTDs.[70] If a vibrating tool, such as a chain saw, is held in an awkward position for prolonged periods, the elbow and shoulder joints are subjected to static loading, and may contribute to premature development of CTDs.[71] Moreover, because of the weight and the need to control a vibrating tool, the worker will tend to grip the tool very tightly. As a result, various tissues of the hand and arm are likely to resonate at certain critical frequencies. This may contribute to degeneration or pain in the wrist and elbow joints.

Vibration is known to cause constriction of blood vessels in the fingers, which gives the fingers a white and pale appearance. This action can also cause numbness and swelling of hand tissues and reduce grip strength.[72] Common names for this syndrome include "white fingers, dead fingers, occupational-Raynaud's and vibration syndrome". Furthermore, tasks such as sanding that involve the use of vibratory hand tools, and also require repetitive movements of the wrist, can have an additive stress-effect on the wrist tendons sufficient to cause carpal tunnel syndrome.[73]

Tool-transmitted forces

Tools transmit various kinds of forces to the hand. When these forces are excessive, or located in especially vulnerable parts of the hand, cumulative trauma can result. For example, short-handled pliers can put tremendous pressure on the palm of the hand where blood vessels and nerves are concentrated. The handle digs into the palm, obstructing blood flow (called ischemia) through the ulnar artery.[74] This trauma leads to numbness and tingling in the hand.

Another example of tool-induced trauma is associated with use of an ordinary paint scraper. This tool is frequently used in cleaning operations in the plastics industry. Pushing the scraper causes pressure in the palm of the hand, cutting off the blood flow to the fingers. This can also be caused by a tool handle that is too small for the worker's hand (Figure 24). The tool handle is then supported in the base of the palm, creating pressure on the blood vessels and nerves, which may cause the worker's fingers to turn cold and white.[75]

The backs and sides of the fingers are also particularly sensitive to excessive pressure because the skin is thinner, with less muscle and fat to absorb shock. The continuous use of ordinary scissors as shown in Figure 25 requires exerting some pressure on the back of the fingers after each cut to open the blades. This can lead to nerve problems in the fingers. Furthermore, pressure concentrations on localized skin areas or small joints may cause penetration of the skin, calluses, soreness, and aggravation of joint problems. Sharp ridges like those on many screwdrivers dig into the fingers, causing

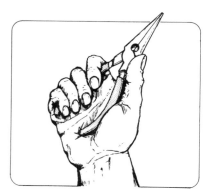

Figure 24. Tool handle that is too short for worker's hand and puts pressure on tissues at the base of the hand.

discomfort and consequently reducing the force that can be applied by the hand.

Using power tools with a bent wrist also increases the risk of a traumatic injury. Because grip strength is significantly less when the wrist is bent, power tools can be more easily dislodged from the hand as a result of a sudden torque or jolt. To compensate for the reduction in grip strength arising from the bent wrist posture, a worker may try to maintain control of the tool by increasing applied grip force which accelerates muscle fatigue.

Human variation

Tools typically have been designed with a specific work population in mind. As the workforce expands and diversifies, there are, however, greater individual differences in workers' physiques, not only between the sexes, but among races and different age groups. Hence, tools that are the right size for one group may be incorrect for another. Furthermore, many hand tools are not designed to accommodate left handed persons, who make up more than 15% of the work population. For example, drills with handles or serrated knives that are usually beveled only on one side result in left-handers applying pressure to the wrong side of the knife and tearing rather than cutting.

Although form-fitting handles, found frequently on power tools, may look as though they fit the hand, they, in fact, are only molded to an average-size hand. What may be good for the average size hand becomes very uncomfortable for a person falling well below or above the average. Unless the handle matches the contours of the user's hand, the handle's finger ridges cause the fingers to separate and reduce the forces that can be applied.

Sex differences are a major source of human variation to be considered in tool design. In a survey of on-the-job complaints from 1400 Air Force women, the two tool-related problems from which most complaints arose were **hand length and grip strength**.[76] The average hand length of the Air Force women was more than 2 cm (0·8 in.) shorter than that of the average male. Furthermore, grip strength of women is on the average two-thirds that of men. If one uses data on maximum power grip for industrial workers, the average woman would have an available strength of about 27 kg (60 lbs) and the average man about 45 kg (100 lbs).[77] An interesting sidelight of this study was that no correlation occurred between the strength of the hand grip and the development of injuries.

Clothing and personal equipment

The amount of clothing and personal equipment a worker uses on the job adds to the effects of human variation. When operating a certain tool, workers may be expected to wear gloves, and gloved hand size is significantly different from ungloved hand size. For example, a glove that fits poorly will alter what was a properly designed hand tool for an ungloved hand into a potentially harmful tool for a gloved hand. Gloves that are too thick also affect the worker's grasp by spreading the fingers

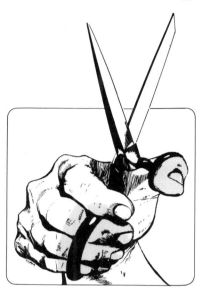

Figure 25. Contact forces between the sides of the fingers and the scissors handles can cause digital neuritis and corresponding numbness and tingling in the shaded area of the hand.

too far apart. Gloves may also interfere with the sense of tactile feedback causing the worker to grip tools more tightly than necessary. The static forces that develop in the tendons of the hand, forearm, and elbow are likely to contribute to the build up of local muscle fatigue and pose a risk of CTDs. Moreover, with a slippery or dry glove, the worker may also over-grip simply to get a firm hold on the tool or parts that have smooth surfaces.[77] Even the use of rubber gloves results in a 15–20% reduction in power grip strength.[78,79] Improper glove sizing may also inhibit the performance of precision control tasks.

Conclusion

Methods were described for determining whether a worksite has employees who have CTDs, or are at risk for developing CTDs. In the absence of reliable medical records, a job analysis may be needed to determine if a cumulative trauma hazard exists. The main point was that **CTD may develop when the work demands habitually exceed a worker's capacity to respond to those demands**. The solution is to **balance work demands with worker capacity**. Methods for achieving this balance are discussed next.

References—Part II

1. Anderson, C.K., Fine, L.J., Herrin, G.D. and Sugano, D.S., 1985, Excess days lost as an index for identifying jobs with ergonomic stress. *J. Occup. Med.*, **27**(10), 740–744.
2. Westgaard, R.H. and Aaras, A., 1984, Postural muscle strain as a causal factor in the development of musculo-skeletal illnesses. *Applied Ergonomics*, **15**(3), 162–174.
3. World Health Organization, 1977, *International System for the Classification of Disease* (Geneva: World Health Organization).
4. Hymovich, L. and Lindholm, M., 1966, Hand, wrist, and forearm injuries: The result of repetitive motions. *J. Occup. Med.*, **8**(11), 573–577.
5. Warwick, D.P. and Lininger, C.A., 1975, *The Sample Survey: Theory and Practice*. (New York: McGraw-Hill Co.).
6. Berdie, D.R. and Anderson, J.F., 1974, *Questionnaires: Design and Use*. (Metuchen, NJ: Scarecrow Press, Inc.).
7. Corlett, E.N. and Bishop, R.P., 1976, A technique for assessing postural discomfort. *Ergonomics,* **19**(2), 175–182.
8. McMurtry, R.Y., Youm, Y., Flatt, A.E. and Gillespie, T.E., 1978, Kinematics of the wrist; Part II: Clinical Manifestations. *J. Bone and Joint Surg.,* **60**(A), 955–961.
9. Phalen, G.S., 1966, The carpal tunnel syndrome. *J. Bone and Joint Surg.,* **48A**(2), 211–228.
10. Drury, C.G., 1983, Task analysis methods in industry. *Applied Ergonomics,* **14**(1), 19–28.
11. Drury, C.G., 1987, A biomechanical evaluation of the repetitive motion injury potential of industrial jobs. *Seminars in Occupational Medicine.* **2**(1), 41–49.
12. Anderson, J.A.D., 1972, System of job analysis for use in studying rheumatic complaints in industrial workers. *Ann. Rheum. Dis.,* **31**, 226.
13. Barnes, R.M., 1980, *Motion and Time Study, Design and Measurement of Work*. (New York: John Wiley), 7th ed, pp. 16–21.
14. Gilbreth, F.B., 1912, The present state of the art of Industrial Management. *Transactions of the ASME.* **34**, 1224–1226.
15. Armstrong, T. and Kochar, D., 1982, Work performance and handicapped persons. In: *Industrial Engineering Handbook*, edited by G. Salvendy. (New York: John Wiley).

16. Barnes, R.M., 1980, *Motion and Time Study, Design and Measurement of Work.* (New York: John Wiley), 1983, 7th ed, p. 117.

17. Last, J.M., 1983, *A Dictionary of Epidemiology.* (New York: Oxford University Press), p. 93.

18. Konz, S., 1979, *Work Design.* (Columbus, Ohio: Grid Publishing, Inc.), pp. 58–60.

19. Eastman Kodak Company, Human Factors Section, 1983, *Ergonomics Design For People at Work* (Vol. I). (Belmont, CA: Lifetime Learning Publications).

20. Grandjean, E., 1980, *Fitting the task to the Man: An Ergonomic Approach.* (London: Taylor & Francis, Ltd), pp. 351–355.

21. Cailliet, R., 1977, *Soft Tissue Pain and Disability.* (Philadelphia, PA: F.A. Davis Co.), pp. 9–12,

22. Armstrong, T.J., Chaffin, D.B. and Foulke, J.A., 1979, A methodology for documenting hand positions and forces during manual work. *J. Biomechanics,* **12,** 131–133.

23. Neviaser, R.J., 1983, Painful conditions affecting the shoulder. *Clin. Orthop. North Amer.,* **173,** 63–69.

24. Wilson, J.R. and Grey, S.M., 1984, Reach requirements and job attitudes at laser-scanner checkout systems. *Ergonomics,* **27**(12), 1247–1266.

25. Steiner, C., 1976, Tennis elbow. *J. Amer. Osteop. Assoc.,* **75**(6), 575–581.

26. Hymovich, L. and Lindholm, M., 1966, Hand, wrist, and forearm injuries: the result of repetitive motions. *J. Occup. Med.,* **8**(11), 573–577.

27. Tichauer, E.R., 1966, Some aspects of stress on forearm and hand in industry. *J. Occup. Med.,* **8,** 63–71.

28. Armstrong, T.J., Foulke, J.A., Joseph, B.S. and Goldstein, S.A., 1982, Investigation of cumulative trauma disorders in a poultry processing plant. *Am. Ind. Hyg. Assoc. J.,* **43**(2), 103–116.

29. Napier, J.R., 1941, The prehensile movements of the human hand. *J. Bone and Joint Surg.,* **38B**(4), 902–913.

30. Ayoub, M.M. and Lo Presti, P., 1971, The determination of an optimum size cylindrical handle by use of electromyography. *Ergonomics,* **14**(4), 509–518.

31. Rogers, S.H., 1987, Recovery time needs for repetitive work. *Seminars in Occupational Medicine,* **2**(1): 19–24.

32. Armstrong, T.J., 1986, Ergonomics and cumulative trauma disorders. *Hand Clinics,* **2**(3), 553–565.

33. Comaish, S. and Bottoms, E., 1971, The skin and friction: Deviations from Amonton's laws and the effects of hydration and lubrication. *Br. J. Dermatol.,* **84,** 37–43.

34. Armstrong, T.J., Chaffin, D.B. and Foulke, J.A., 1979, A methodology for documenting hand positions and forces during manual work. *J. Biomechanics,* **12,** 131–133.

35. Swanson, A.B., Matev, I.B. and de Groot, G., 1970, The strength of the hand. *Bull. Pros. Res.,* **10,** 145–153.

36. Hertzberg, H.T.E., 1955, Some contributions of applied physical anthropology to human engineering. *Annals of the New York Academy of Sciences,* **63**(4), 616–629.

37. Tichauer, E.R., 1966, Some aspects of stress on forearm and hand in industry. *J. Occup. Med.,* **8**(2), 63–71.

38. Silverstein, B.A., Fine, L.J. and Armstrong, T.J., 1986, Hand, wrist cumulative trauma disorders in industry. *Br. J. Ind. Med.,* **43,** 779–784.

39. Armstrong, T.J., Fine, L.J. and Silverstein, B.A., 1985, Occupational Risk Factors: Cumulative Trauma Disorders of the Hand and Wrist. *Final Report on NIOSH Contract* No. 200–82–2507 (Cincinnati, OH: NIOSH).

40. Ohara, H., Nakagiri, S., Itani, T., Wake, K., and Aoyama, H., 1976, Occupational health hazards resulting from elevated work rate situations. *J. Human Ergol.,* **5,** l173–182.

41. Cafarelli, E., Cain, W.S. and Stevens, J.C., 1977, Effort of dynamic exercise: Influence of load, duration and task. *Ergonomics,* **20**(2), 147–158.

42. Basmajian, J.V. and De Luca, C.J., 1985, *Muscles Alive: Their*

functions Revealed by Electromyography, 5th edition (Baltimore MA; Williams & Wilkins), pp. 201 and 290.

43. Maeda, K., 1977, Occupational cervicobrachial disorder and its causative factors. *J. Human Ergol.,* **6,** 193–202.

44. Bjelle, A., Hagberg, M. and Michaelson, G., 1981, Occupational and individual factors in acute shoulder-neck disorders among industrial workers. *Br. J. Ind. Med.,* **38**(4), 356–363.

45. Rohmert, W., 1973, Problems in determining rest allowances. Part 1: Use of modern methods to evaluate stress and strain in static muscular work. *Applied Ergonomics,* **4**(2), 91–95.

46. Chaffin, D.B., 1973, Localized muscle fatigue—definition and measurement. *J. Occup. Med.,* **15**(4), 346–354.

47. Corlett, E.N. and Bishop, R.P., 1978, The ergonomics of spot welders. *Applied Ergonomics,* **9**(1), 23–32.

48. Borg, G., 1971, The perception of physical performance. In: *Frontiers of Fitness* edited by R. J. Shephard (Springfield, IL: Charles C. Thomas), pp. 280–294.

49. Armstrong, T.J., Radwin, R.G., Hansen, D.J. and Kennedy, K.W., 1986, Repetitive trauma disorders: Job evaluation and design. *Human factors,* **28**(3), 325–336.

50. Hunting, W., Laubli, T.H. and Grandjean, E., 1981, Postural and visual loads at VDT workplaces — I. Constrained postures. *Ergonomics,* **24**(12), 917–931.

51. Hunting, W., Laubli, T.H. and Grandjean, E., 1980, Constrained postures of VDU operators. In: *Ergonomic Aspects of Visual Display Terminals*, Proceedings of the International Workshop, Milan, March 1980, edited by E. Grandjean and E. Vigliani. (London: Taylor & Francis), pp. 175–184.

52. Bhatnager, V., Drury, C.G. and Schiro, S.G., 1985, Posture, postural discomfort and performance. *Human Factors,* **27**(2), 189–199.

53. Grandjean, E., 1982, Postural Research. In: *Anthropometry and Biomechanics Theory and Application*, edited by R. Easterby, K.H.E. Kroemer and D.B. Chaffin. (New York: Plenum Press).

54. Corlett, E.N., 1983, Analysis and evaluation of working posture. In: *Ergonomics of Workstation Design*, edited by T.O. Kvalseth. (London: Butterworths), pp. 12–15.

55. Chaffin, D.B., 1973, Localized muscle fatigue: Definition and measurement. *J. Occup. Med.,* **15,** 346–354.

56. Hagberg, M., 1984, Occupational musculoskeletal stress and disorders of the neck and shoulder: A review of possible pathophysiology. *Int. Arch. Occup. Environ. Health,* **53,** 269–278.

57. Rohmert, W., 1973, Problems of determination of rest allowances. Part 2: Determining rest allowances in different human tasks. *Applied Ergonomics,* **4**(3), 158–162.

58. Herberts, P. and Kadefors, R., 1976, A study of painful shoulder in welders. *Acta Orthop. Scand.,* **47,** 381–387.

59. Das, B. and Grady, R.M., 1983, Industrial workplace layout and engineering anthropology. In: *Ergonomics of Work Station Design,* edited by T.O. Kvalseth. (London: Butterworths), pp. 103–128.

60. Diffrient, N., Tilley, A.R., Harman, D. and Bardagjy, J.C., 1981, *Humanscale: 1,2,6 and 7* (Cambridge, MA: MIT Press).

61. Das, B. and Grady, R.M., 1983, The normal working area in the horizontal plane — A comparative analysis between Farley's and Squires' concepts. *Ergonomics,* **26**(5), 449–459.

62. Armstrong, T.J., Radwin, R.G., Hansen, D.J. and Kennedy, K.W., 1986, Repetitive trauma disorders: Job evaluation and design. *Human Factors,* **28**(3), 325–336.

63. Ayoub, M.M., 1973, Work place design and posture. *Human Factors,* **15**(3), 265–268.

64. Ridder, C.A., 1959, *Basic Design Measurements for Sitting.* (Agricultural Experiment Station, University of Arkansas, Fayetteville) Bulletin 616.

65. Fraser, T.M., 1980, *Ergonomic Principles in the Design of Hand Tools.* Occupational Safety and Health Series, No. 44. (Geneva, Switzerland: International Labour Office).

66. Tichauer, E.R. and Gage, H., 1977, Ergonomic principles basic to hand tool design. *Am. Ind. Hyg. Assoc. J.,* **38,** 622–634.

67. Williams, N., 1975, Biological effects of segmental vibration. *J. Occup. Med.,* **17**(1), 37–39.
68. Armstrong, T.J., Foulke, J.A., Joseph, B.S. and Goldstein, S.A., 1982, Investigation of cumulative trauma disorders in a poultry processing plant. *Am. Ind. Hyg. Assoc. J.,* **43**(2), 103–116.
69. Charash, R., 1982, Tools need not harm the hands that use them. *Industrial design,* **29,** 42–45.
70. Pelnar, P.V., Gibbs, G.W. and Pathak, B.P., 1982, A pilot investigation of the vibration syndrome in forestry workers of eastern Canada. In: *Vibration Effects on the Hands and Arms in Industry*, edited by A.J. Brammer and W. Taylor. (New York: John Wiley), pp. 173–187.
71. Pyykko, I., 1986, Clinical aspects of the hand-arm vibration syndrome: A review. *Scand. J. Work Environ. and Health,* **12,** 439–447.
72. Farkkila, M., 1978, Grip force in vibration disease. *Scand. J. Work Environ. and Health,* **4,** 159–166.
73. Taylor, W., 1974, *The Vibration Syndrome.* (New York: Academic Press).
74. Tichauer, E.R. and Gage, H., 1977, Ergonomic principles basic to hand tool design. *Am. Ind. Hyg. Assoc. J.,* **38,** 622–634.
75. Tichauer, E.R., 1966, Some aspects of stress on forearm and hand in industry. *J. Occup. Med.,* **8**(2), 63–71.
76. Ducharme, R.E., 1977, Women workers rate male tools inadequate. *Human Factors Society Bulletin,* **20,** 4.
77. Kamon, E., and Goldfuss, A.J., 1978, In-plant evaluation of the muscle strength of workers. *Am. Ind. Hyg. Assoc. J.,* **39**(10), 801–807.
78. Tichauer, E.R. and Gage, H., 1977, Ergonomic principles basic to hand tool design. *Am. Ind. Hyg. Assoc. J.,* **38,** 622–634.
79. Wang, J., Bishu, R. and Rodgers, S., 1983, Data from studies of the effects of gloves on grip strength collected at State University of New York at Buffalo. *Unpublished.*

Part III

Preventing Cumulative Trauma Disorders

Part III of this manual focuses on two strategies for controlling or preventing the occurrence of CTDs. *Instituting personnel-focused work practices* and *Redesigning tools, work stations and jobs*. The merits of each strategy are discussed. Combinations of elements of each strategy are frequently used in workplaces where prevention programs for CTDs have been implemented. A series of guidelines for ergonomic redesign are also provided along with a list of references for further information on ergonomic measures as applied to controlling cumulative trauma hazards.

Administrative and engineering controls

The recommendations for prevention can be conveniently classified as being either primarily **administrative** (focusing on **personnel solutions**) or **engineering** (focusing on **redesigning tools, work stations and jobs**).

Administrative controls refer to those actions taken by the management or medical staff to limit the potentially harmful effects of a physically stressful job on individual workers. Administrative control is achieved by **modifying existing personnel functions** such as worker training, job rotation, and matching employees to job assignments. In other words, the control actions are focused on the worker. This subject is covered in Chapter 8, Instituting personnel-focused work practices.

By contrast, engineering control focuses on the job or work environment. The aim here is to redesign the job or tool to achieve control over those job factors associated with the onset of CTDs. This subject is covered in Chapter 9, Redesigning tools, work stations, and jobs.

Getting approval and support

Regardless of the prevention strategy adopted, it is always necessary to gain the support of key people in your organization, namely: (1) upper management who will have to approve the recommendation for changes, (2) the engineering, safety, and personnel staff who have to implement the changes, and (3) the workers who are affected by the changes.

Furthermore, whatever the proposed plan of control, it will have to be justified. This justification is likely to include a discussion of the extent of the problem, the number and severity of CTD cases and estimates of the time, expense, and disruption involved in carrying out the control program.

In addition to the expected justifications required for approval, it may also be necessary to conduct an educational seminar for the decision or policy makers in the work establishment. These people could include the plant manager, department supervisors and first-line foremen. More than likely, these people are not well informed about CTDs and will need to be briefed for purposes of obtaining their approval and support for carrying out indicated control programs. Specific examples of high-risk jobs from the affected plant should be identified using procedures outlined in Part II of this manual. If possible, some solutions should be proposed along with estimates of costs and benefits.

Two basic methods exist for justifying the need for a control program: social and legal justifications, and economic justifications. The social-legal justifications center around a company's responsibilities to protect its employees against workplace hazards and the fundamental desire to do what is right.*

The economic justifications involve the likely costs of CTDs versus the costs and benefits of preventing them. Such an analysis should center around the possibilities of reduced overhead costs, reduced non-productive time, and improved productivity. Factors involved in overhead expenses and non-productive time might include: medical costs, compensation costs, lost productivity because of injuries and absenteeism (including overtime and increased workforce size to make up for absenteeism) and labor turnover.

Social-legal justifications can sometimes be very effective and should not be overlooked. One approach is to focus on the problems of specific people who are suffering from CTDs. A presentation might sketch out their history with the company, the type of work they do, the kinds of physical problems they are experiencing, the likely course of the disorder, the specific aspects of their work that probably caused the problem and ways in which these factors might be controlled.

Once the approval of key management has been accomplished, it is necessary to develop a plan for effectively mobilizing the support of others in the organization. Of course, the details of the plan will depend on the unique characteristics of the workplace, but a few basic points can be made:

(1) Give the people you will be relying on as much knowledge and information as possible.

---

*U.S. Occupational Safety and Health Act of 1970. Sec. 5 (a) Public Law 91-596. "Each employer shall furnish to each of his employees employment and a place of employment which are free from recognized hazards that are causing or are likely to cause death or serious physical harm to his employees" . . .

(2) Be frank about problems that exist and about what you do and do not know.

(3) Do not force your ideas on others, though you may have more expertise concerning CTDs.

(4) Come to the workers with an open mind and do not talk down to them.

(5) Recognize that those who carry out the work, both workers and supervisors, often have the best ideas on how things might be changed to satisfy particular objectives.

(6) Give workers a real opportunity to be involved in the planning and implementation of changes that affect them.

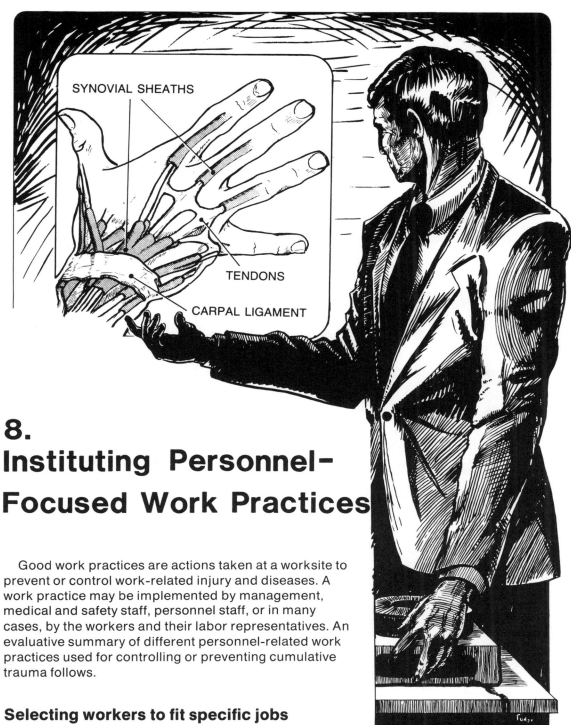

SYNOVIAL SHEATHS

TENDONS

CARPAL LIGAMENT

8.
Instituting Personnel-
Focused Work Practices

Good work practices are actions taken at a worksite to prevent or control work-related injury and diseases. A work practice may be implemented by management, medical and safety staff, personnel staff, or in many cases, by the workers and their labor representatives. An evaluative summary of different personnel-related work practices used for controlling or preventing cumulative trauma follows.

Selecting workers to fit specific jobs

No valid methods exist yet for accurately predicting whether healthy workers are susceptible to CTDs before hiring. Attempts to screen potential employees through wrist X-rays, muscle strength tests, tests of physical fitness or flexibility, or other means have not proved successful and may be viewed as discriminatory.* Moreover, the courts

---

*U.S. Federal Rehabilitation Act of 1973, and 44 states have laws that prohibit discrimination in employment.

have deemed that it is management's responsibility to show the relevance of its screening test in identifying minimum and essential attributes needed by workers to safely and effectively perform the job.

The success of any screening program ultimately depends on obtaining accurate information as to the specific **demands of the job**. An accurate assessment of worker capacities is also needed, particularly as it relates to key job demands. Any assessment of human capacities is complicated by the influence of a variety of psychosocial factors including work performance, motivation, expectation, and fatigue tolerance.

For example, it is generally accepted that muscular strength is an appropriate job-related criterion for a variety of manual jobs including construction, heavy assembly, packing/shipping, etc. If a job analysis indicates that the essential requirement for the job is sufficient upper body strength, then an appropriate strength test must be designed. The ideal test must accurately simulate the force, frequency, and endurance demands inherent in the main components of the job.

Criteria are also needed for deciding the level of a worker attribute that is necessary to meet the job demands. For example, if the results from a pre-employment test indicate that two candidates are equal except for strength, who should be hired? Is the weaker worker a poor risk? There are no defensible guidelines yet for such decisions.

A secondary aim of worker selection might be to assign people to jobs according to their physical stature. A tall worker, for example, might be able to comfortably reach the top of a machine or part, whereas a much shorter one would have to exert added force with the arms held above the shoulder level. A short worker, on the other hand, might have the advantage of working at benches that would be too low for some. Selecting workers according to stature may prove acceptable if there are sufficient numbers of workers available who fit the workstation or task requirements. Certainly this approach could not be used in conjunction with a worker rotation schedule.

These examples highlight the need for developing **minimum acceptability criteria** to avoid the tendency to hire only the strongest or youngest workers. Selecting workers for strength or size opens the door to possible abusive discrimination. For example, size and strength are both correlated with sex. Worker selection for strength or size may unwittingly discriminate against women and older employees.

In summary, attempts to determine the strength or dexterity demands of a job, and the relative strength and dexterity of workers, is a complex process because of the wide variety of physical job demands inherent in the workplace, the range of individual physical capacities, and the lack of criteria for safely and effectively matching workers to jobs.

Finally, some companies use a system called bidding-for-jobs. When a job becomes available, interested workers may sign up for it. The worker with the most seniority gets the job. This essentially eliminates management's role in assigning workers to particular jobs, and it would eliminate the viability of worker selection as a control technique for CTDs. Some self-selection would occur to avoid highly stressful jobs, particularly for those workers with CTDs.

A safety and health department staffed by personnel able to assess both the human performance capacities and the demands of the various jobs in their plant can perhaps make judicious decisions about worker selection. But a foreman or department manager who must juggle a constantly changing workforce during the first minute or two of each work day, and who may not fully understand the hazards involved in various jobs, may not be able to practice successful worker selection. Unless the immediate supervisors thoroughly understand what is involved in worker selection, they are likely to unintentionally undermine any attempt to use this method for CTD control.

Training workers

To train workers in the prevention of CTDs is to teach them to work efficiently in a safe and healthful manner. This generally involves training aimed at reducing the number and types of awkward wrist, arm and shoulder postures, minimizing the levels of mechanical forces applied, and reducing the number of repetitive motion patterns. Simply telling workers about the risk factors that can contribute to CTDs and advising them to avoid engaging in those behaviors would appear to be a straightforward matter. The essential question, however, is one of the effectiveness of such instruction.

Training is providing someone with a needed skill. Informing someone about the general factors involved in CTDs, and recommending that they avoid those behaviors, **may make that person aware that something needs to be done differently**. It may not, however, give them any idea about how their job should be done.

Even if specific information is provided to the worker about how a job can be done to avoid CTDs, the worker may still be unable to do the job in the recommended way for any number of the following reasons:

(1) The accustomed way of doing things may be an ingrained habit.
(2) There may be production pressures to take short cuts.
(3) The new way may be more difficult or more time-consuming.
(4) The threat of developing CTDs may seem remote.
(5) The work process, (job layout as designed) may not permit the prescribed actions needed to reduce the trauma risk factors.
(6) The weight and shape of the materials handled are usually beyond the worker's control.

Training principles

The first step in training is to clearly specify the objectives — that is, one must know exactly what behaviors are to be taught.

This can be accomplished by closely watching or analyzing a videotape of someone doing the job. By studying the videotapes, potentially hazardous work postures and movements can be identified. Criteria for identifying work patterns that are biomechanically unsound can be obtained from guidelines appearing in this manual and in standard ergonomic reference texts cited at the end of this manual. After identifying the problems or conditions that you seek to change through training, it is advisable to do the job yourself (incorporating the training objective) to make sure that you understand what is involved and that the recommended changes can be followed.

Communicating the objectives consists of showing or telling the trainees what you want them to do. Manual skills are generally easier to communicate by allowing someone to observe the recommended way of doing things, either by a live demonstration or a videotaped or filmed presentation. A minute or two of demonstration can be worth thousands of words.

Ideally, a trainee should have an opportunity to practice a recommended skill immediately after it is shown. The immediacy of the opportunity minimizes the chances of forgetting. On-the-job practice is the most realistic. Appropriate feedback can be given to correct faulty performance.

Much industrial training is conducted with little thought as to whether or not the learned behaviors can be easily maintained after training. For example, a worker may be better protected from CTDs if he occasionally uses a particular tool in carrying out a specific task. The worker may be given the tool and trained in its use. However, if there is great pressure to keep up a particular pace of work, or if using the new tool requires extra time and effort, the effects of the training will probably not endure.

Before embarking on a course that requires particular work behaviors, make sure that, (1) there are no work pressures or demands that would impose restrictions on those behaviors, and (2) the work environment will support those behaviors. If the CTD control program requires support from an immediate supervisor who is always pushing production instead of encouraging healthful work habits, it is to be expected that maintaining the objectives of the training will be difficult. An appeal to upper level management may then be necessary.

Efforts are under way in some industries to broaden training beyond the fundamental issues of safe work practices and to include more comprehensive approaches, such as (1) hazard recognition programs for increasing worker awareness and (2) problem-solving programs designed to provide workers with the information and skills necessary to participate in hazard control activities.

Training conclusions

Although industrial training programs are easy to implement and have an intuitive, rational appeal based on the belief that behavioral change follows awareness, their success in reducing CTDs has been mixed. A second reason for the interest in training is that it is usually less costly than ergonomic interventions. Experience has shown, however, that over the course of a few years, the costs of on-going training programs may exceed the initial expenses needed to implement ergonomic changes in the job or tools used. A main reason for the continuing expense of training programs is that each new employee must be trained, and retrained periodically to reinforce safe work practices.

Training programs have traditionally focused on teaching employees specific work practices for safety and hygiene. Though most experts support such training, the actual effectiveness of such programs has been difficult to evaluate. More recently, the concepts of training have been extended to include elements of recognition and problem solving. Moreover, it is now recognized that training, or more appropriately, **education aimed at awareness** is needed at all levels of management, including such staff specialists as loss-control personnel, procurement officers and engineers who are concerned with tool and workplace design and use.

Worker rotation

The purpose of rotating workers from one job to another is to reduce the duration of exposure of any one worker to tasks that call for stressful postures, forces, and highly repetitive activities involving the arm, wrist, and hand. Worker rotation schemes are complicated by the fact that no one knows with certainty what is an acceptable exposure to a cumulative trauma causal factor.

Worker rotation may also pose an increased hazard of injury. For example, a worker may lack experience with the rotated jobs and suffer what is called **response interference**. An example of this was found in a food processing plant where workers were rotated from fish filleting to trimming operations. Both jobs required the use of a knife, but filleting required high force, whereas trimming required small precise motions. Workers who rotated between the two jobs had difficulty adjusting to the different forces needed and ended up over-cutting or under-cutting. This increased their risk of suffering severe finger or hand cuts.

Worker rotation may also violate certain employment agreements or collective bargaining issues governing job assignments. Supervisors may also object to worker rotation because of the need to maintain consistent production levels. For example, worker rotation may disrupt the supervisor's job assignments that place the most highly productive or skilled employees on the more demanding jobs. Obviously, the supervisor's cooperation is necessary, and more important, their understanding of the intent of the job rotation is necessary.

The purpose of using worker rotation as a control for CTDs is to help alleviate physical fatigue and stress by systematically alternating job demands and task duration by rotating workers through different jobs. However, if a worker is rotated into what appears to be a different job —but in reality imposes the same physical demands as the previous job —worker rotation will fail to achieve the goal of alleviating physical fatigue and may even accelerate the condition.

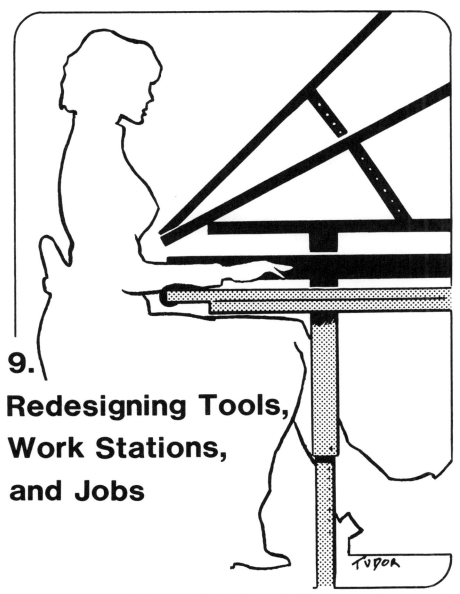

9.
Redesigning Tools, Work Stations, and Jobs

Once a job analysis has established the probable source of the cumulative trauma, a plan for control and prevention should be devised. The preceding section outlined three personnel-focused work practices used to control the incidence of CTDs. The conclusion was that training, job rotation and worker selection represent "people" solutions to what are essentially job design and equipment problems. Hence, such administrative procedures should only be considered as temporary measures to be used until a more permanent solution is available. A permanent solution is one in which safe work is a natural result of the design of the job, workstation and tools, and is independent of specific worker capabilities or work techniques.

Changing the job, not the worker

The guiding principle of this section is **to make the job fit the person, not to make the person fit the job**. This goal is accomplished by redesigning the job or tool to reduce the job demands of high force, repetition, and awkward postures.

Ultimately, by improving the fit between the worker and the job, we are not only contributing to the well-being of the worker, we are also improving productivity. We call this the **ergonomic solution**.

Ergonomics is an applied science concerned with the design of workplaces, tools, and tasks to match the physiological, anatomical, and psychological characteristics and capabilities of the worker. Ergonomics as a discipline draws from the fields of physiology, anatomy, psychology and engineering for theory and methodology.

Special skills and training are needed to design and implement changes in jobs, tools, and work methods. Experts in this field usually have had formal training in one or more of the following areas: industrial and biomechanical engineering, work physiology, anatomy, applied psychology and industrial hygiene.

Coping with obstacles in redesigning jobs

Often the initial task of identifying the causes of CTDs is overshadowed by the more difficult task of deciding on the most effective method of control or intervention. There is seldom a simple, single change to be made. More often there are numerous overlapping problems involving some combination of high production demand, faulty work methods, awkward workstation layouts, or ill-fitting tools. Furthermore, what may be an effective ergonomic intervention for controlling cumulative trauma at one workplace may be totally inappropriate at a sister plant with a different work population. Perfect solutions are rarely available and design decisions often involve compromises and trade-offs.

There is also the risk that a proposed ergonomic solution, like any therapeutic regimen, may have a side effect that outweighs the proposed benefit. For example, providing a chair may alleviate lower back and leg fatigue, but may increase the distance the operator has to stretch to reach certain controls or supplies. Hence, attempts to alleviate one source of cumulative trauma may create or contribute to new injuries or illnesses that may even be more serious than what is being remedied.

Perhaps the most cautious way to proceed is to administer an ergonomic intervention with the same degree of care as one would use with any new remedy. One should:

(1) Perform a thorough examination first (job analysis) to determine the specific problem.
(2) Evaluate and select the most appropriate intervention(s) (the assistance of an expert may be useful here).
(3) Start conservative treatment (implement the intervention), on a limited scale if possible.
(4) Monitor progress.
(5) Continue to adjust or refine the scope of the intervention as needed.

Despite the potential difficulties associated with the development and implementation of any type of intervention or control program, there remains a pressing need to provide some practical guidelines for redesigning jobs that carry risks of CTDs.

What follows is a discussion of the principles and recommendations of ergonomic experts on the prevention of CTDs.

Design principles based on ergonomics

The majority of the guidelines presented in this manual for achieving ergonomic control over cumulative trauma have one or more of the following three objectives:

(1) Reduction of extreme joint movement.
(2) Reduction of excessive force levels.
(3) Reduction of highly repetitive and stereotyped movements.

Reduction of extreme joint movement

Since excessive stress on joints and tendons is a principle cause of CTDs, motions that are performed often should be kept well within the range of motion of that joint. Work activities should ideally be performed with the joints at about the midpoint of their range of movement. When force is being applied by the hand, the wrist should be kept straight and the elbow bent at a right angle. All side-to-side deviations of the wrist should be avoided. The hands should be kept in line with the forearms.

At least three methods exist for reducing deviations of the wrist:

(1) **Altering the tool or controls**
(e.g. bending the tool or handle instead of the wrist)
(2) **Moving the part**
(e.g. rotating the part in front of the worker so the wrist can be straight)
(3) **Moving the worker**
(changing the position of the worker in relation to the part)

Reduction of excessive force

Since tasks requiring prolonged and excessive muscle contractions to maintain a posture (or to assemble a part, or hold an ill-fitting tool) contribute to the development of CTDs, jobs should not require the worker to exert more than 30% of his or her maximum force for a particular muscle, **in a prolonged or repetitive way**. All muscular contractions, including occasional ones, in excess of 50% of the maximum should be avoided.

Exertion level or fatigue can also be minimized by heeding the relationship between load and duration. Simply, decreasing the required effort (load) by as little as 10% will allow work to continue at a constant level for a period that exceeds the original duration by a factor of five or six. In essence, work fatigue is influenced more by load than duration. The ratio of load to duration may be as high as 10:1, respectively.

Available charts and tables provide a general range of strength for specific muscle groups in men and women of different age groups and worker stature.[1,2]

Three general approaches to controlling job forces are:

(1) **Reducing the force required** (keep cutting edges sharp,

use weaker springs in triggers, power with motors rather than muscles, use jigs and clamps instead of hands to grip parts.
(2) **Spreading the force** (use trigger levers rather than single-finger push buttons and allow the worker to alternate hands).
(3) **Getting better mechanical advantage** (use stronger muscle groups and use tools with longer handles).

Reduction of highly repetitive movements

Since highly repetitive and stereotyped manual movements contribute to CTDs, potentially aggravating production and design factors must be identified and altered to reduce the repetitive levels of a work cycle. Counter-measures include limiting the duration of continuous work or restructuring of work methods.

Although it is difficult to define repetition levels that can be labeled as always harmful, jobs that have a cycle time of less than 30 seconds and a fundamental cycle that exceeds 50% of the total cycle time, should be considered as posing a risk for CTDs. A fundamental cycle is a work cycle that has a sequence of steps or elements (Therbligs) that repeat themselves within the cycle.

Several approaches may be taken to reduce rates of repetition:

(1) **Task enlargement**. Restructure jobs so that each worker has a larger and more varied number of tasks to perform. This must include a corresponding increase in job-cycle-time.
(2) **Mechanization**. The use of special tools with ratchet devices or power drivers can reduce stressful repetition.
(3) **Automation**. Repetitive tasks are performed best by a machine. To be cost effective, this must typically involve a high-volume, long-term production process.

Design of work stations

Given the opportunity, most employees will begin to customize their work area to enhance efficiency or reduce some aspect of fatigue. If they share the work area with others, the extent of any customizing will be limited to items that a worker may bring to work or that can be quickly installed and removed when work is finished. For example, workers may bring special seat cushions to compensate for height variations when chair or stools are not adjustable. Special mats, rugs, or even make-shift risers may be used to stand on to reduce shoulder fatigue from working with arms raised. Crates may be placed on benches by tall workers to reduce bending of the shoulder and neck. Some creative employees may even rearrange the location of their supplies and output bins for disposing of waste and finished products.

Supervisor reactions to such worker initiatives are varied. Some may object if changes interfere with the work of others or with the department's overall productivity or safety. Other supervisors may even encourage or seek advice from workers regarding needed improvements. However, the criterion for deciding what job modifications are actual improvements may rest solely on productivity and thus fail to reduce sources of cumulative trauma to the worker.

From the above examples, it can be seen that improvements in workplace design are usually the result of trial and error. The purpose of this section is to provide some guidelines based on ergonomic principles for planning the layout or modifications of work stations to **minimize the stressful effects of repetitive and static work patterns**.

Guidelines for work stations[3]

Design work stations to accommodate different people

An ergonomic work station should accommodate a vast majority of the people who work on a given job and not merely the average. A work station that is adjustable and was either designed or selected to fit a specific task should be experienced as relatively comfortable by 90% to 95% of the worker population. The work space should also be large enough to accommodate the full range of required movements. For the seated operator, certain space requirements should be observed. Minimum requirements are given in Figure 26a and b.

Data for design decisions can come from a variety of sources:

(1) **Anthropometric tables** offer extensive listings of the size measurements and proportions of the human body as distributed in the adult population, and are especially

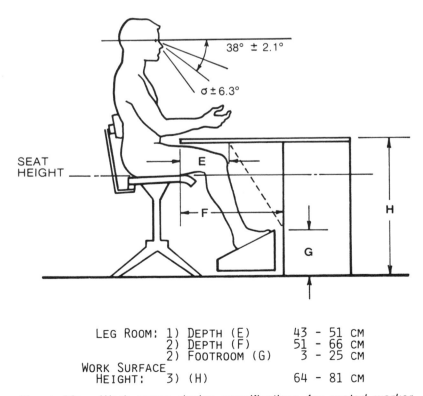

```
 LEG ROOM:  1) DEPTH (E)       43 - 51 CM
            2) DEPTH (F)       51 - 66 CM
            2) FOOTROOM (G)     3 - 25 CM
 WORK SURFACE
      HEIGHT:  3) (H)          64 - 81 CM
```

Figure 26a. Work space design specifications for seated worker (adapted from Ayoub, 1973.)[4]

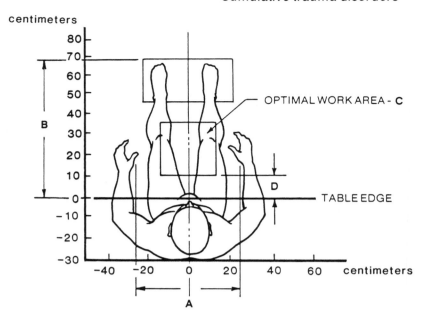

LEG ROOM: 1) WIDTH (A)   MINIMUM OF 50 CM
             2) DEPTH (B)   65 CM, IF LIMITED
OPTIMUM WORK AREA: 3) (C)   APPROXIMATELY 25 X 25 CM
             4) (D)   10 CM FROM EDGE OF WORK SURFACE

Figure 26b. Work space design specifications for seated worker (adapted from Ayoub, 1973.)[4]

helpful at the drawing board stage of a new work station. (See NASA Source Book, 1978, and the Humanscale series by Diffrient *et al.*, 1981)

(2) **Fitting trials** use actual workers in an inexpensive cardboard mock-up of a possible work station. This mock-up trial allows for adjustments of key dimensions for each subject so that an optimum final design may be made.

(3) **Fatigue measurements** in the laboratory and factory involve using scientific instruments to measure muscle activity and force.

Permit several different working positions

To avoid static loading of muscles, good work station design should permit the worker to adopt several different but equally healthy and safe postures which still allow performance of the job. Ideally, a worker should be able to choose either a sitting or standing position. Arm rests and foot rests should be supplied when appropriate.

An example of work stations at which a worker can either sit or stand are shown in Figure 27. Notice that the shape of the tool handle may have to be changed to maintain a neutral wrist position when the worker assumes different positions. This example illustrates one of the difficulties in designing multipurpose work stations for seated and standing postures, and the accompanying need to fit the tool to the worker's different postures to reduce stressful wrist deviations.

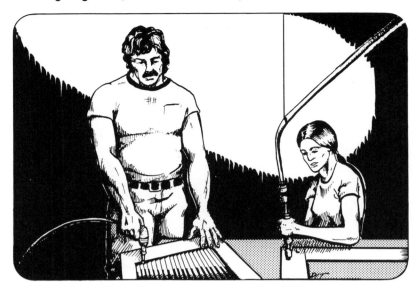

Figure 27.   *Shows the effects of being seated or standing on the type of tool handle needed to maintain a straight wrist.*

Whether a worker should be standing or sitting depends on the type of task to be performed. Sitting is best for tasks that require fine precision work. This position requires less muscle activity to maintain the posture and provides greater stability for the worker. Foot controls can also be operated more easily. Standing is best for tasks that require a large space to be covered or large forces to be exerted.

Design should start from the working point, where the hands spend most of their time

Frequent work should be kept within the area that can be conveniently reached by the sweep of the forearm, with the upper arm hanging in a natural position at the side of the trunk. The area that can be reached by extending the arm from the shoulder will vary greatly, depending on the size of the worker.

If the worker has to use the hand to grip an object, the maximum reach of the arm should be reduced by 5 cm (2 inches) or more. An occasional stretch to reach beyond this range is permissible since the momentary effect on shoulders and trunk is transient. However, if this becomes a permanent part of a job, forearm or shoulder fatigue may be experienced. In general, the design should allow the worker to maintain an upright and forward-facing posture during work. Figure 28 provides a graph layout of average reach distances for wrist, thumb and finger tips for both sitting and standing.

Place controls, tools, and materials between shoulder and waist height to be easily reached and manipulated

Avoid reaching above shoulder level or behind the body. All reaching should be below and in front of the shoulder. There should be a definite and fixed space for all tools and materials. Their location should be close to the point of use, and they should be arranged so that they permit the best sequence of motions. Figure 29a illustrates a worker using a punch press

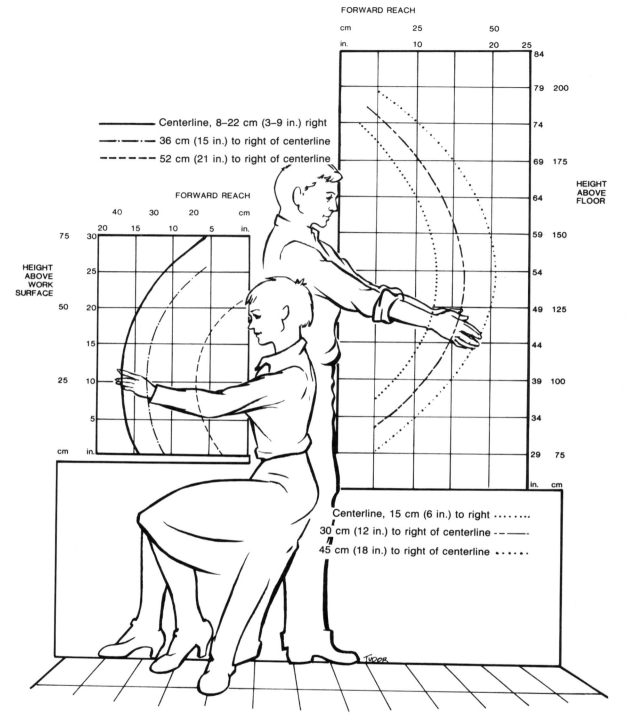

Figure 28.   Graphic aid for estimating reach distances for sitting or standing (average worker).

where the controls are located overhead requiring extreme shoulder elevation. An improved version is illustrated in Figure 29b where the controls were moved away from the press and relocated at waist level. Figure 30 illustrates acceptable and unacceptable work areas for positioning repetitive work with respect to the hands and arms. If the surface height is too high, the arms are held away from the body (abducted) and static loading of the shoulder muscles results.

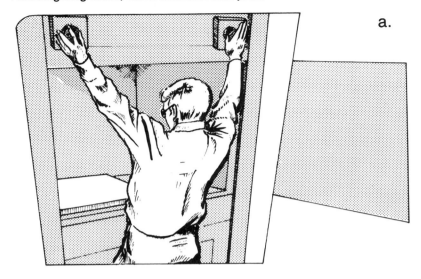

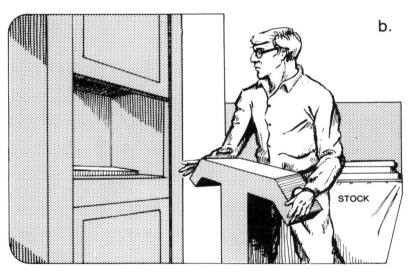

Figure 29. *Example of workplace redesign showing relocation of punch press controls to waist level to reduce need for overhead arm extension, while keeping hands safe.*

The more precise the work, the higher the work surface. The heavier the work, the lower the work surface

As a general rule, for most types of industrial jobs, the work area should be about 5 to 10 cm (2–4 in.) below the elbow when standing or seated in an erect posture. This is measured with the elbows held close to the body and arms bent at 90 degrees. The arm should hang from the shoulder in a relatively relaxed position allowing the forearm to be nearly horizontal.

In addition to using the worker's elbow height as a guide for setting the height of work surfaces, the force requirements of the task should also be considered. For example, the work area may be raised 5 to 10 cm (2–4 in.) above the elbow for very precise or delicate work, whereas for heavy manual-assembly jobs, the work surface should be 10–15 cm (4–5 inches) below elbow height. For jobs where the work surface is elevated above elbow

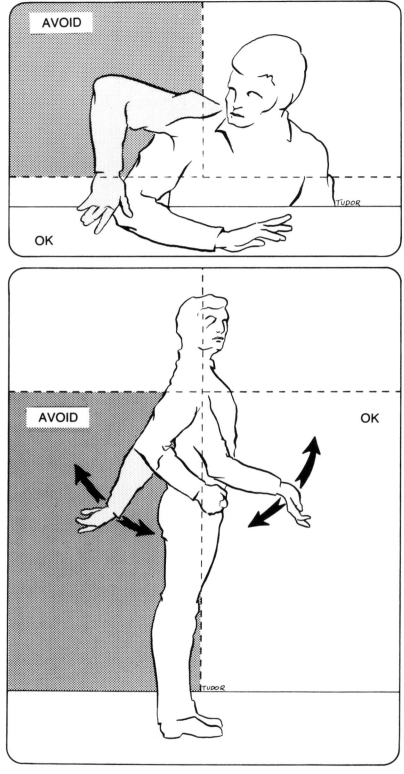

Figure 30.   Arm and elbow positions to be avoided and positions that are acceptable (OK) for repetitive jobs.

height, adjustable pads should be provided for resting the forearms.

The optimal work surface height for the seated worker is more complicated because it is a function of the height of the seat or chair, the thickness of the work surface and the worker's thigh. Figure 31a and 31b show a set of recommendations for work surface heights based on the type of work performed for both the seated and standing worker, respectively.

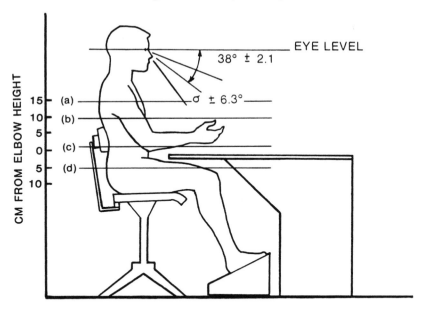

a. For fine work, exacting visual tasks
b. For precision work, e.g., mechanical assembly work
c. For writing or light assembly work
d. Coarse or medium manual work such as packaging

Figure 31a.   Design specifications for correct height of work surface for seated operator (adapted from Ayoub, 1973).[4]

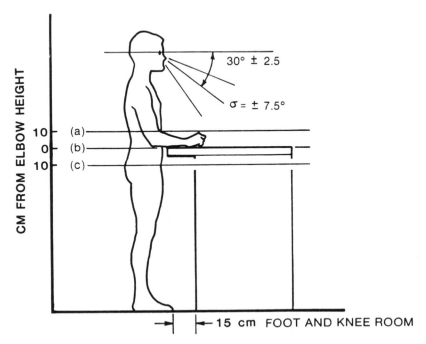

a. For precision work with supported elbows
b. For light assembly work
c. For heavy work

Figure 31b.   Design specifications for correct height of work surface for standing operator (adapted from Ayoub, 1973).[4]

All edges of the work surface should be well rounded and
padded where an elbow or forearm might be rested

Figure 32a depicts a worker's elbow supported on the surface
of a work bench to stabilize the hands and rest the shoulders.
This posture places pressure on the ulnar nerve and in time can
produce numbness and tingling in the fingers. Stresses on the
elbow can be reduced by cushioning and rounding the edge, as
in Figure 32b.

Provide well-designed chairs

Make sure the chair is correctly designed for the job and the
person. Despite the fact chairs and stools have been used in
workplaces for years, there has been remarkably little attention,
until recently, to the design or selection of chairs that actually fit
the job or the worker. A chair that is inappropriate is not only a
source of discomfort, which can affect productivity, but in the
long run can contribute to back, neck, and leg problems.

One of the impediments to good chair design has been the
erroneous notion that sitting is a static activity, when in fact, it is a
dynamic one. People need to be able to move around in their
seats, lean this way and that, and get up and down easily.
Moreover, seating should be viewed in relation to the worker's

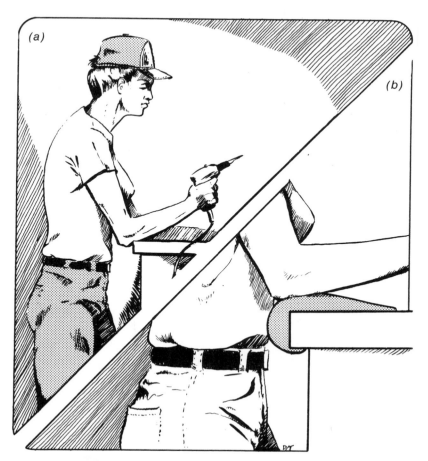

Figure 32(a).   A work posture that places pressure on the ulnar nerve.
(b) A rounded pad placed over the edge of the work table relieves
pressure on the ulnar nerve as it passes over the elbow.

task. Since chair comfort is task-dependent as well as person-dependent, there is seldom a single chair that will satisfy the needs of all workers. The seat height, back rest, and foot rest should be adjustable to accommodate 90% of the population and the adjustments should be simple and easy to perform.

A methodology for evaluating chairs has been developed using a combination of fitting-trials and user comfort-evaluation.[5] The report also provides a "chair-feature checklist", that is useful for individuals needing to evaluate chairs for industrial or office use.

An example of an adjustable chair with both arm and lumbar support is shown in Figure 33.

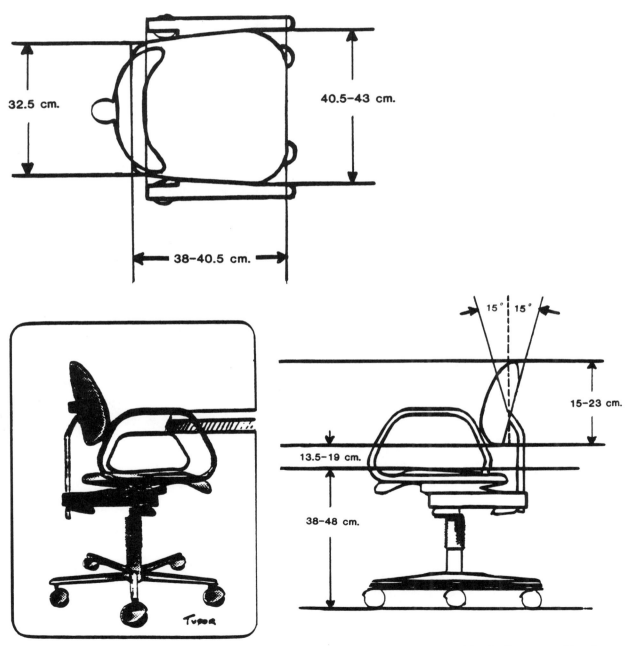

Figure 33.   Example of an adjustable chair with design specifications that provides both arm and lumbar support.

GUIDELINES TO PROPER CHAIR DESIGN AND FITTING ARE:[6,7]

(1) Inclusion of a small kidney-shaped backrest, which provides mobility and support. Position the backrest to clear the pelvis to ensure maximum mobility.

(2) Chair height should be adjustable so that work surface is slightly below elbow height. If the seat is too high, legs will dangle, increasing pressure on the underside of the thighs. If the seat is too low, knees will be raised, putting leg muscles under tension.

(3) Clearance must be provided for thighs. The distance between the top of the seat and bottom of the work surface should be 29–30 cm (about 11 inches).

(4) Footrests may be useful for high chairs or short people. Position the footrest to take weight off the thighs. A good footrest offers a large surface on which to place the feet.

(5) Position both the seat depth and the back rest to avoid pressure at the back of the knee (the popliteal cavity). The seat front should be rounded to eliminate pressure in the popliteal area, which contains nerves and blood vessels.

(6) Provide arm rests if they do not interfere with necessary movement. Often one arm rest on one side will suffice.

(7) The seating surface should be slightly slanted backwards (3 to 5 degrees) to prevent sliding out of the seatpan and encourage the use of a backrest.

(8) The seat should be upholstered with a slightly porous, rough-textured material that does not give way more than 2–3 cm.

Design of work methods

Every job has a set of procedures for accomplishing the work. The origin of these procedures usually can be traced to the need by management to plan the staffing requirements for the new job. For example, information is needed to determine how long the job will take, what skills or physical demands are required of the worker, and what is the optimal method or sequence of motions for performing the job. To obtain such data, a work-methods analysis is often conducted (see Part II, Chapter 7).

Despite the fact that traditional work methods analyses were designed primarily to obtain staffing and production estimates, work-methods analyses can provide useful information for identifying the physical stress to the hands, arms, and shoulders that contribute to CTDs. For example, by closely examining the Methods–Time Measurements system (MTM) coding, and with a sketch of the workplace, the durations of both static holding postures and repetition rate can be computed.

Traditional work-methods analysis, however, does not provide needed information on force levels or on hand and arm postures. Hence, job analyses conducted to identify sources of cumulative trauma require an additional assessment of the actual load or force applied by the workers. Although force may be assessed using electromyographic techniques, the procedure is too cumbersome and time consuming for routine work analysis. One alternative is to use a psychophysical procedure to assess the worker's level of perceived exertion.

The most widely used is the Borg Rating of Perceived Exertion (RPE) scale. In general, measures of perceived exertion or effort correlate highly with objective measures of work load, such as heart rate.[8,9]

Appendix A of this Manual defines and illustrates a variety of stressful postures and terms used to describe them.

Guidelines for redesigning work methods

The following guidelines were developed largely from experience with job analysis, including MTM, and from experience with the application of ergonomic principles to job redesign. A few of the more time-tested guidelines that have been used to control sources of cumulative trauma in the workplace are presented.

Use jigs and fixtures whenever possible

Many jobs are performed with the non-preferred hand acting as a "biological jig" because no other means of holding the work piece is provided. An example of a useful fixture for holding a typewriter housing is shown in Figure 34. The top half of the figure (a) shows the original wrist posture in which the worker must flex her wrist and exert pressure to hold a sander against a typewriter housing. In the bottom half of the figure (b), an adjustable fixture is shown for holding and orienting the part. The sander handle has also been redesigned to reduce the wrist flexion.

Duck-billed pliers fastened at an appropriate height and actuated by a pneumatic or hydraulic cylinder serve as convenient jigs for holding small parts that would otherwise demand a pinch grip by the operator.

Jigs for complex items can be produced cheaply with quick-setting plastic, which can be molded to hold unusual shapes. A slightly oversized part or movement of the part during the molding operation will ensure that parts can be easily put into the plastic jig and removed at the end of the cycle. Jigs and products should be designed for easy assembly. Lead-ins for holes and tool-entry points reduce assembly time and reduce the need for static loading of the operator at the entry point. Figure 35 illustrates two jigs, (a) and (b), which required the operators to bend their wrist. An improved version is shown in (c).

Re-sequence jobs to reduce repetition

Analyze the sequence of elements to see where both long static contractions and frequent repetitions occur. Both should be avoided. Often the element sequence can be rearranged to break up a long static contraction or to spread repetitions across both hands.

For seated operators, a foot pedal may be used to activate a jig or to eject a work piece from a jig. When analyzing the manual sequence of motions, determine whether alternative muscle groups may be brought into use for highly repetitive elements. This will distribute the work load over different muscle groups and joints.

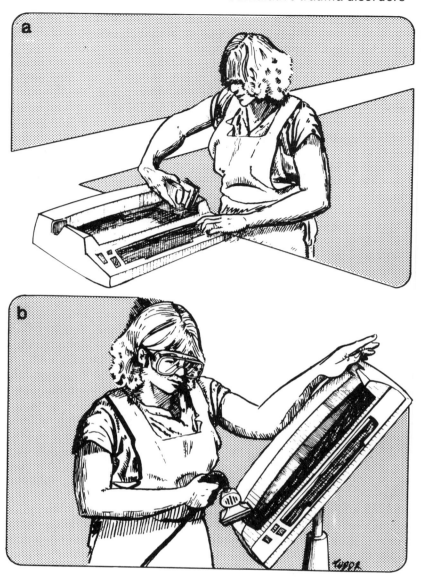

Figure 34. *Example of a jig (b) that corrects for faulty wrist posture shown in (a).*

JIGS

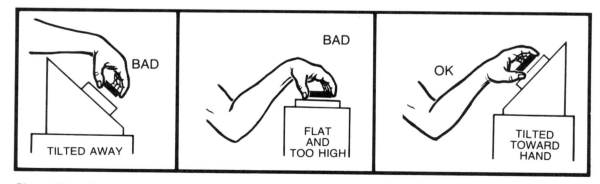

Figure 35. *Jigs should be located and oriented so that parts can be assembled without flexing the wrist.*

Combine jobs to reduce repetition

In addition to reorganizing work methods within a cycle, thought should be given to reassigning tasks to operators as a method of reducing repetition rates. This means combining jobs that had previously been broken down to provide very short cycle times with each movement being repeated many thousands of times per day. Often, combining jobs can also lead to reduced materials handling, reduced storage for work in progress and reduced unpacking and repacking of containers.

Industrial relations researchers have found that job design has the added benefit of increasing job satisfaction and worker productivity. Enlarged jobs not only reduce the degree of repetition by increasing the cycle time and diversity of manual activity but they can also provide the worker with a sense of accomplishment.

Feelings of accomplishment stemming from job enlargement provide the worker with a greater sense of personal control and responsibility for a finished product. Job enlargement or enrichment, as it may be called, is a viable alternative to job rotation. Moreover, it may improve worker productivity in ways that worker–job rotation cannot.

Combining jobs means that for the same output, more parallel work stations may be needed. Hence if a particular machine or tool is required for one operation, more machines or tools will often be needed, and they may not be used all of the time. CTDs, however, are rarely associated with complex and expensive machines that need to be run for 24 hours a day to be profitable. Rather, CTDs occur predominantly in industries such as sewing, small parts assembly and meat preparation, where tools and machines are simple, have a lifetime far beyond their payback period, and may be used for one or two shifts per day. In general, the costs of CTDs far outweigh the costs of purchasing additional tools and machinery for parallel work stations.

Automate highly repetitive operations

Because of the complex nature of work procedures in some plants, it may be too difficult or costly to redesign certain jobs to eliminate the stressful biomechanical elements of work. Under these conditions, automation or semiautomation may be required. By using robotic techniques, engineers can eliminate many high-risk jobs and substitute machines to take over these stressful tasks while the operator performs the remaining tasks. This technology has recently been introduced in the automotive industry, where robots perform jobs that are hazardous and highly repetitive in nature, such as welding, painting, and finishing. However, automation can also have negative side effects. While it has relieved the worker from performing many of the more strenuous and dangerous jobs, it has also served to simplify jobs, often reducing them to single repeated acts that focus the biomechanical forces on smaller, more vulnerable parts of the musculoskeletal system, such as the hands and wrist.

Allow self-pacing of work when possible

Most of the studies supporting this recommendation provide only general statements indicating that one work condition, such as paced work, causes more or less work strain than another, e.g., non-paced work.[10,11] A fixed pace is only optimal for a small percentage of workers. For the majority of workers, a fixed pace may be either too slow to provide adequate challenge to hold their attention and maintain work motivation, or alternately, a fixed pace may be too fast to allow sufficient recovery between work cycles to prevent local muscle fatigue. Hence, any work design that provides the worker with some control over the pace will make it easier to find people who will not only do the job, but remain on the job.

New employees should start at a slower rate

By starting at a slower pace an employee can become **work hardened** or conditioned prior to assuming full work capacity. A few hours of warm-up may only be needed for a conditioned worker, whereas several weeks may be needed for a worker returning from an injury or CTDs. Just as athletes recognize the need for conditioning and stretching to increase muscle efficiency and coordination, and to prevent injuries, workers who are introduced to the job at a slower pace develop improved work practices and are less likely to experience start-up soreness. Soreness is attributed in part to micro-tears in the connective tissue in response to forceful lengthening from unaccustomed repetitive exertions. The degree and extent of conditioning should be tailored to each worker's capacity and the demands of the job.

Allow frequent rest pauses

Rest pauses should be scheduled to **provide relief for the most active muscles** of the upper extremity used in the job. By contrast, most conventional notions concerning rest pauses are designed to conserve the worker's overall workload (energy expenditure). Usually, a work:rest ratio is determined by assessing the duration of heart rate recovery.

By comparison the guideline offered here is based on worksite experience indicating that the incidence of upper extremity CTDs is more a function of the work and rest of the forearm and intrinsic hand muscles than of overall work load.[12] Guidelines for estimating rest pauses for repetitive jobs involving various levels of effort, based on maximum voluntary contractions (MVC), can be obtained from inspection of the graph shown in Figure 36. To use this graph, job information is needed on the **effort required**, and on either the **total cycle time**, or **holding time**. If the job is externally paced, the cycle time is known. The holding time can be obtained with a stop-watch from videotapes of the job. To estimate effort, a simple rating scale has been devised that corresponds to the MVC.[13] From this scale effort is categorized into one of the three levels shown on the graph: light, moderate, or heavy.

The needed recovery time for a given level of effort is determined from the graph and, depending on the available information, either the cycle time or holding time is used as starting point. A straight line is drawn from either the cycle time or holding time values to intersect with the appropriate effort level. Another line is then extended back to the coordinate axis. **Recovery time is equal to the total cycle time minus the holding time for a given level of effort**. For example, an overhead

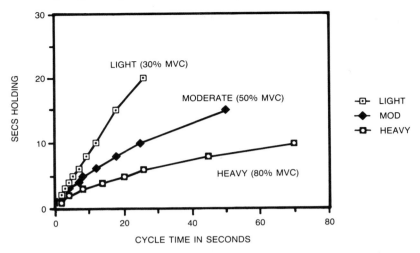

Figure 36. *Work and recovery guidelines, adapted from data in Rohmert[13] and Rodgers[19].*

assembly task, categorized as heavy, that has a 30 second cycle time (paced at 120 insertions per hour) should, based on the graph, require no longer than a 6 second holding time to complete one insertion cycle. The minimum recovery time is then 24 seconds.

Although this model is based on limited data collected some years ago,[14] it does provide a simple method for assessing the need for task redesign either to shorten hold time, reduce effort levels, or increase total cycle time (which would reduce the work pace). Additional research on work/recovery is needed not only to verify the existing model, but also to provide more precise measures of work effort.

In summary, the above three guidelines all involve the issue of time, i.e., pacing, work rates, work duration and recovery. A main difficulty in obtaining this type of data is the specificity of each work situation and the difficulty in making generalizations from one job task to another. A second problem rests with the accepted criterion as to what is a realistic work schedule that meets the goals of the company and still provides the workers with a margin of protection against overuse and exertion injuries. In general, guidelines for work duration, rest breaks and production levels need to be derived directly at the work site for each job situation. This should be evaluated in terms of the protection afforded to the workers, which is often a process of trial and error.

Design of tools and handles[15]

Tools and handles increase man's productivity by extending and amplifying manipulative abilities. Since productivity is associated with a worker's livelihood, workers are motivated to carefully select and in some cases customize their own tools when given the opportunity. Moreover, proper attention to the selection and design of tools and workstation layouts can minimize the risk of CTDs.

Until recently, few guidelines were available to help workers select tools that were both effective and safe to use. Workers relied on trial and error procedures to find the right tool for the job. The right tool was judged not only on its effectiveness, but also by how it felt, the balance, and its weight, shape, and handle size. Hence, an effective tool not only aids productivity, but also minimizes the development of fatigue and physical stress that accumulates over the course of a work day. Fortunately, these two criteria can be made compatible by applying principles from the field of ergonomics. Tool and handle design for preventing CTDs rests on four fundamentals:

(1) **Avoiding high contact forces and static loading**
(2) **Avoiding extreme or awkward joint positions**
(3) **Avoiding repetitive finger action**
(4) **Avoiding tool vibration**

The following guidelines are offered for the design and selection of tools and handles. The guidelines were derived from numerous studies conducted over the last 15 years, and they include recommendations covering hand tools, power tools and container handles.

Guidelines for selecting and designing tools

Handles should be provided[16,17]

Handles are essential. Many tools are designed so that the operator must grasp a motor housing or an air cylinder rather than a handle. This exposes the hand to vibration, cool air currents from the motor, skin compression and abrasion from contact with the tool surface, and skin burns. A properly designed tool handle should isolate the hand from contact with the tool surface, enhance tool control and stability, and serve to increase the mechanical advantage while reducing the amount of required exertion.

Design for minimum muscular effort

To operate a hand tool at least one hand must support it in place and apply some type of leverage (or pressure on a switch). Both support and control require static muscular contractions in the arm and fingers, a process which is fatiguing. Ideally, the support function should be separated from the application of force and control.

The workstation layout should also be designed so that between work cycles, the tool can either be conveniently laid down or inserted into a holster. Otherwise, consider suspending the tool overhead using retractor linkage. Various types of suspension systems and counterweights are available for holding tools. A tool that weighs between 4 kg (10 lb) and 6·5 kg (15 lb) cannot be held by the forearm in a horizontal position for more than 2 or 3 minutes without experiencing extreme muscle discomfort.

Since finger muscles are small and individual muscle groups are relatively weak, even small forces may exceed a worker's maximum force capacity. Similarly, if a hand grip is too small or too large, these weaker muscles are working at a disadvantage.

The center of gravity of the tool should be located close to the body to reduce fatigue. Heavy or unbalanced tools will tire the muscles very quickly, particularly if the arm must be extended outward. Handles should also be located close to the tool's center of gravity to reduce the tendency of the tool to slip out of the hand.

Power with motors more than with muscles

Whenever possible, power tools should be used to reduce the amount of human force and repetition required. In some cases a simple ratchet mechanism can greatly reduce hazardous repetitive motions. Careful attention should also be paid to selecting a power tool of minimum weight and making sure the operator has a minimum length of power cords and lines to contend with. Some brands of power tools are twice as heavy as others with identical power outputs and equal reliability records. There are some exceptions to the principle of selecting the lightest tool; these are discussed on page 108.

Bend the tool, not the wrist

This principle is illustrated in Figure 37. On the left side of this figure, a hand is shown gripping conventional pliers that cause an ulnar deviation. An improved version of the pliers with a bent handle is shown on the right side of Figure 37. This version allows the wrist to maintain a neutral position. The actual degree of bend in the tool depends on the task performed and the workplace layout. The Western Electric bent-pliers have a 35-degree bend; soldering irons can have a 90-degree bend; and hammers have been designed with a 5 to 15 degree bend.

Assembly operations typically require the use of powered-hand tools to drive screws. To control the tool rotation or torque, workers must often use grip forces that may be near their maximum strength capacity. If the proper tool or handle shape is

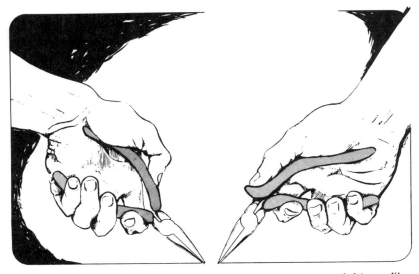

Figure 37. The straight pliers on the left have a straight profile requiring an ulnar deviation of the hand when working at bench level, whereas the bent pliers on the right allow the worker to maintain the wrist in a neutral position.

not used, the worker may add to his or her biomechanical stress by **bending the wrist into awkward postures** to complete the assembly. Figure 38 illustrates this problem and the potential solution for a motorized screw-assembly task. Two types of drivers are shown in Figure 38 — the cylindrical, in-line handle and the pistol grip driver. The handle of the pistol grip is bent between 70–90 degrees. Figure 38 serves to emphasize the point that it is the orientation and location of the work pieces relative to the position of the worker that dictates the choice between tool shapes.

In general, tools with pistol grips should be used where the tool axis must be horizontal. A straight grip should be used where the tool axis is vertical, or where the direction of force is perpendicular to the work plane. Straight tools can be purchased with removable pistol grips to reduce tool inventory and maintenance costs and still accommodate the operator.

The use of specialized tools, such as the bent-handle tools, are most effective in applications where (1) all of the work is

POWERED DRIVERS

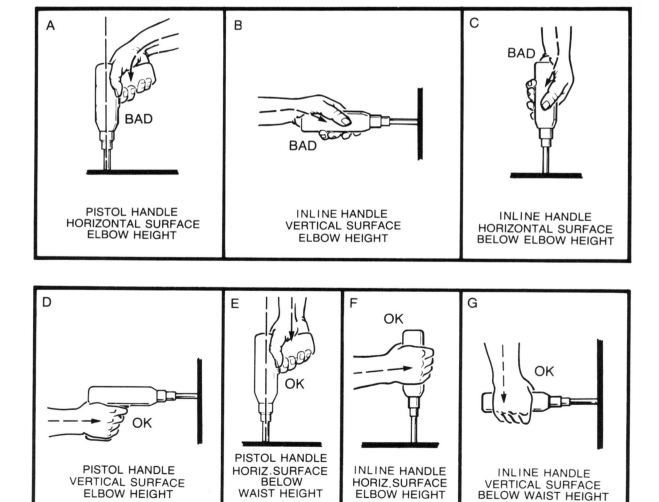

Figure 38.   Example of wrist postures used with various hand tools and work station layouts. [18]

done in the same plane (i.e., horizontal or vertical), and (2) only one or two other tools are used. Jobs where frequent switching between specialized tools are required will contribute to increased operator fatigue and slowed production. In such cases, consider designing a single tool with multiple uses that encourages the use of neutral postures.

Avoid tool designs that require the wrist to be flexed and the arm pronated at the same time, as this stretches the tendons and may contribute to lateral epicondylitis (tennis elbow). In addition to wrist deviations, wrist flexions or extension, extremes of elbow flexion and shoulder abduction contribute to the stress on tendons and nerves of the hand.

Finally, avoid the use of tools that require flexion of the last joints on the finger, the distal phalanges. If trigger movements are needed, design the movement so that both the middle and end sections of the fingers can be bent simultaneously. As a rule use a trigger strip as opposed to a trigger button. This reduces local finger muscle-fatigue while increasing force capacity. The index finger and second finger can be combined and used to activate a trigger (Figure 39).

Keep the weight of the tool low

In repetitive tool usage, the weight of the tool should be kept low because of the high frequency of use. Workers should be able to easily hold the tool with one hand. Tools heavier than 0·5–1 kg (1–2 lbs) should be supported by a counter-balancing harness. [Also see page 104 — the use of minimum muscular effort.]

The tool's center of gravity should also be aligned with the center of the grasping hand. Arm muscles should not have to correct for improper tool balance. An example of a tool that is front heavy is the typical electric drill shaped like a gun. Maintaining proper tool balance will also keep the hand from being whipped around by rotational tool movements or torque.

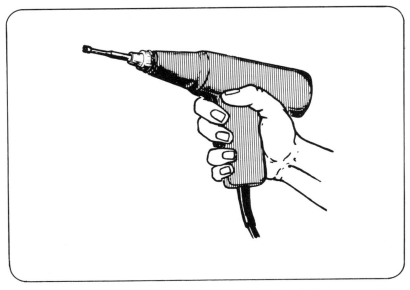

Figure 39. Example of a tool with a trigger that is long enough to accommodate 2 or 3 fingers.

When applied to power tools there are some exceptions to this principle of "low-tool-weight". Specifically, if a power tool is too light, the operator has to provide the force and often must grip harder and add shoulder tension to the task, increasing the risk of CTD problems. For example, a grinder or buffer needs a certain amount of weight to provide sufficient inertia to prevent transmission of vibration to the hands and arms and to provide even pressure on a surface.

Use special-purpose tools

Adapt the tool to the task rather than having the operator adapt to a general-purpose tool. For example, where power tools are needed to tighten both horizontal and vertical fasteners on an assembly, it may be possible to combine two tools into one to perform two functions so that the operators do not have to change tools as frequently. If a job is causing CTD problems, it will usually be cost effective to redesign tools with the specific job and workers in mind.

Standard off-the-shelf tools are rarely ideally suited to a particular task, but they are easy to modify. It will usually be economically feasible to design special handles. Examples would be the scissors used in the sewing industry or special knives used for butchering poultry.

Design tools to be used by either hand

The majority of commercially available manual tools are designed for the typical right-handed worker. Examples are electrical circular saws, industrial power sanders and scissors. Tools should be symmetrical or easily altered for use by left- and right-handed people. Those that are not adaptable create difficulties for left-handed people and discourage the alternate use of the non-preferred hand to avoid awkward positions, or to allow relief of the hand.

Use a power grip for power and a precision grip for precision

Handles and hand grips should generally be designed for a power grip, in which the hand wraps around the handle. The power grip is capable of generating more force than other grips. Handles that allow a power grip are less fatiguing because they require a lower percentage of the worker's total gripping strength to maintain control of the tool.

For maximum precision in aiming and placing a tool, a precision grip is used. This can be either the internal precision grip (gripping a carving knife) or the external (holding a pencil). Regardless of type, a precision grip should be avoided, particularly for jobs that are intensive and of long duration. Muscle groups involved in precision grips are usually not used to their greatest mechanical advantage, which accelerates the onset of fatigue. The pinch grip requires large muscle and tendon forces relative to the force produced. It is inefficient and fatiguing and should be avoided in any engineering effort to control CTDs.

Make the grip the proper size and shape

The most common error in handle design involves providing handles that are too small. One reason is the belief that smaller tools should have smaller handles. The other common problem, particularly with large tools is the use of a handle that is too large in diameter (e.g., when the worker is expected to use the motor housing of a tool as a handle).

Handles and grips should be cylindrical or oval with a diameter of between 30 mm and 45 mm (1·25–1·75 in.).This diameter improves grip and control of the tool without sacrificing torque capacity. For precision operations, a diameter ranging from 5 mm to 12 mm (0·2 to 0·5 in.) is recommended.

Flutes or ridges may be provided on the handle of tools such as screw-drivers if high torque ability is required. However, if these ridges and flutes are very deep or have sharp edges, they often cause excessive pressure on the soft tissues of the palm. Textured rubber handles will usually provide enough friction for a good grip. A small diameter and smooth front end on a tool will also allow better control and manipulation. A T-shaped handle provides greater torque with less grip force.

The minimum handle length for any tool is 100 mm

Since the average worker's hand or palm is about 100 mm (4 in.) across, a 100 mm handle is the absolute minimum for handle length. In order to provide the worker some freedom of hand placement on the handle, a 115 mm–120 mm (5 in.) handle is preferable, if it does not interfere with other design considerations. For tools that are used with gloves, add 10 mm (0·5 in.) to the handle length.

Handles that are too short do not allow all of the fingers to grip. As a result, the handle may dig into the palm, pressing on nerves and reducing blood flow. Such tissue compression-stress should be avoided. If a handle must be tightly grasped or squeezed, the handle should be well rounded to allow the forces to be distributed over as large an area as possible.

If high force is required, it should only be applied to large, insensitive, and non-critical areas of the hand. It is particularly important to avoid heavy pressure on the center of the palm. Moreover, the force output should provide enough sensory feedback during the task to allow the operator to provide the correct amount of pressure.

Use handle spans appropriate for men and women

For tools with a handle span (e.g., pliers), the recommended maximum distance between the two handles is between 50 mm and 67 mm (2·0–2·7 in.) for both men and women. The span over which a power grip is exerted will influence how much strength is available for the task. Grip spans that are either too small or too large change the type of grip used. For example, if the grip is too small for the hand, the worker may use a pinch grip, which reduces the worker's effective grip-strength by approximately 25%.[19]

Avoid form-fitting handles

Form-fitting tool handles, such as those often found on pistol grips of power tools or handles on heavy-duty pliers, should be matched carefully with the population intended to use them. Though handle finger-grooves may look as though they were molded to the hand, they are in fact only molded to one particular size of hand. What gives good utility to a person with an average hand becomes very uncomfortable for a person with an exceptionally large or small hand. If the fingers are stretched to fit form-fitting features of hand tools, power is lost and the ability to operate the instrument is impaired. This happens because it is difficult to flex the fingers while they are held apart.

Spring load pliers and scissors

Tools such as metal snips require the operator to exert pressure against the metal handle to open the jaws, causing calluses and trauma to the soft tissues on the back and sides of the hand. A provision of an automatic spring-opening on tools such as scissors and pliers will enable the operator to use strong hand-closing muscles rather than weak hand-opening muscles. An example of a spring-loaded scissors is shown in Figure 40. Opening the jaws by means of a finger inserted between the handle induces a cramped posture of the hand and may also cause trigger finger. Where the operator must exert a force along the handle, as in pushing on a pump screwdriver, a large rounded finger guard at the forward end of the handle will also help reduce the grip forces required.

Provide larger triggers

Triggers on power tools should be at least 51 mm (2·0 in.) so they can be activated by 2 or 3 fingers. Trigger strips will reduce the stresses on the first finger and allow other modes of operation. If a one-finger trigger is used, allow enough room for the whole hand to grip the tool with the finger off the trigger and outside the trigger guard. This arrangement prevents inadvertent operation of the tool when it is being carried. With a handle longer than 55 mm (2·2 in.), the operator may have difficulty relaxing his or her grip without losing control of the tool (see Figure 39).

Relief from static loading can be obtained if the operator can momentarily release the tool by relaxing the grip. A strap around the back of the hand can help, like the grips on ski poles. With a strap, a tool can be held correctly for re-grasping and the grip force can be relaxed between operations. However, if more than one tool is used at the work station, a strap around the grip will interfere. In that case, each tool should have its own tool holder or be counterbalanced on an overhead hanger so that it can be released and re-grasped easily.

Tool handles should be non-porous, non-slip, and non-conductive

Glossy paint or highly polished surfaces on tools should be avoided. A material such as rubber or plastic will avoid the absorption of chemicals and be resistant to small chips and grit

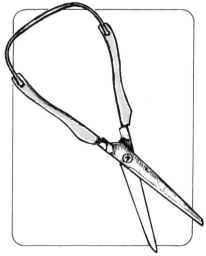

Figure 40. Spring-loaded scissors that prevent irritation of the backs and sides of the fingers caused by opening conventional shears.

while providing good heat and electrical insulation. Grasping surfaces should be slip resistant.[20] As an alternative to wearing gloves a new type of porous safety-tape is now available that has a rubberized coating to preserve the frictional characteristics of the fingers and allow sweat evaporation.

Special absorbent sleeves are also commercially available for fitting over tool handles (Figure 41). The sleeve consists of an outer layer of leather-like plastic and an inner layer foam plastic, all held on the tool by a fabric fastener. Compressible rubber handles provide enough friction for a good grip and are superior to metal flutes or ridges. Although rubber sleeves will not attenuate vibration frequencies much below 700 Hz, they do reduce the amount of force exerted on the tools.

Finally, tool handles should not conduct electricity or heat. Heat-conductive handles (usually metal) can become hot with the heat dissipated from an electric motor or, more commonly, cold because of expansion of compressed air in an air tool. A cold conductive handle reduces hand temperature, a condition associated with the aggravation of a number of CTDs.

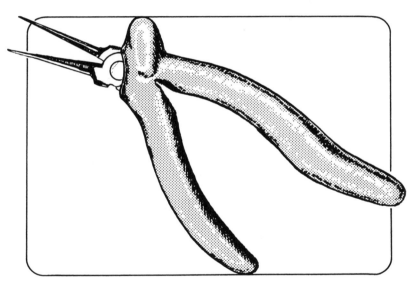

Figure 41. Western Electric pliers with compressible plastic coated handles. The handles are spring-loaded to open automatically.

References—Part III

1. Diffrient, N., et al., 1981, *Humanscale 1–4*. (Cambridge, MA: MIT Press)
2. *NASA Anthropometric Source Book*, Vol. I and II, 1978, edited by Webb Associates. (Washington, D.C.),Pub.No. 1024.
3. Corlett, E.N., 1978, *The Human Body at Work: New Principles for Designing Work Spaces and Methods*. Management Services, May 1978.
4. Ayoub, M.M., 1973, Work place design and posture. *Human Factors,* **15**(3), 265–268.
5. Drury, C.G. and Coury, B.G., 1982, A methodology for chair evaluation. *Applied Ergonomics,* **13**(3), 195–202.
6. Mandal, A.C., 1981, The seated man (Homo Sedens). *Applied Ergonomics,* **12**(1), 19–26.
7. Koffler Group, Ergonomics in the Office Environment, 1983, *The Ergonomics Newsletter.* **2**(1), 1–26.

8. Borg, G., 1971, Psychological and physiological studies of physical work. In: *Measurement of Man at Work,* edited by W.T. Singleton, J.G. Fox and D. Whitfield. (London: Taylor & Francis Ltd.), pp. 121–128.

9. Stamford, B.A., 1976, Validity and reliability of subjective ratings of perceived exertion during work. *Ergonomics,* **19**(1), 53–60.

10. Kuorinka, I., 1981, Work movements in semi-paced tasks. In: *Machine Pacing and Occupational Stress,* edited by G. Salvendy and M.J. Smith. (London: Taylor & Francis Ltd.), pp. 143–149.

11. Smith, M.J., Hurrell, Jr., J.J. and Murphy, Jr., R.K., 1981, Stress and health effects in paced and unpaced work. In: *Machine Pacing and Occupational Stress,* edited by G. Salvendy and M.J. Smith. (London: Taylor & Francis Ltd.), pp. 261–267.

12. Rodgers, S.H., 1987, Recovery time needs for repetitive work. *Seminars in Occupational Medicine,* edited by S.H. Rodgers, **2**(1), 19–24.

13. Borg, G.A.V., 1982, Psychophysical bases of perceived exertion. *Med. Sci. Sports Exercise,* **14**(5), 377–381.

14. Rohmert, W., 1973, Problems in determining rest allowances. Part I. *Applied Ergonomics,* **4**(2), 91–95.

15. Greenberg, L. and Chaffin, D.B., 1977, *Workers and Their Tools.* (Midland, MI: Pendell Publishing Co.).

16. Drury, C.G., 1980, Handles for manual materials handling. *Applied Ergonomics,* **11**(1), 35–42.

17. Tichauer, E.R. and Gage, H., 1977, Ergonomic principles basic to hand tool design. *Am. Ind. Hyg. Assoc. J.,* **38**(11), 622–634.

18. Armstrong, T., 1983, *An Ergonomic Guide to Carpal Tunnel Syndrome.* (Akron, OH: AIHA).

19. Jacobsen, C. and Sperling, L., 1976, Classification of the hand grip. A preliminary study. *J. Occup. Med.,* **18**(6), 395–398.

20. Armstrong, T.J., 1985, Mechanical considerations of skin in work. *Am. J. Ind. Med.,* **8,** 463–472.

Summary

Occupational safety and health professionals have become increasingly concerned with the potential for workers who perform certain hand-intensive jobs to develop CTDs.

These disorders, which primarily affect the soft tissues of the musculoskeletal system, are associated with repeated or sustained exertions in awkward or static postures. They may also involve a high concentration of stress in the upper extremities. Examples of CTDs in this category include: tendinitis, tenosynovitis, De Quervain's disease, epicondylitis, carpal tunnel syndrome, and thoracic outlet syndrome.

Although these trauma disorders have historically been known to exist in the workplace, they are only now recognized as a major cause of lost time and human suffering.

Research conducted at various worksites over the last few years confirmed earlier clinical observations that attributed many of the CTDs to improperly designed work surfaces and/or improper selection of tools that place excessive stress on the tendons, muscles and nerves of the upper extremities.

In an occupational setting, the recommended intervention is to **modify or redesign the job or the tool** to minimize sources of biomechanical trauma. Based on the theory that work-related trauma is the principle causal factor, such an action should result in a reduced incidence of occupational musculoskeletal disorders.

In general, it is recommended that jobs should be designed to maintain the wrist in a neutral posture that is neither flexed toward the palm, nor hyper-extended toward the back of the hand, or deviated side-to-side. Also, the elbows should be kept at the sides of the body. Objects that are held in the hands should be designed to distribute the forces over the largest area possible, avoiding contact with areas over the nerves at the sides of the fingers, base of the palm and elbows. Other factors such as force, frequency and vibration should be minimized even though safe levels have not been determined.

It is hoped that the information contained in this manual will help health professionals, workers, and employers be more cognizant of the types of work patterns that have a potential to cause various CTDs and be aware of the types of ergonomic interventions that can be used to reduce these problems at the workplace.

Appendix A:

Terminology for Body Position and Movement

Accurately describing body movements in everyday language is often difficult. For example, to say that someone bends his wrist tells us very little. In what direction? How far? Is the palm facing up or down? Thus, to describe precisely the position and movement of the human body, science has had to develop specialized terminology.

Although this manual uses a minimum of technical language, there are a number of standard terms used in defining various postures and motions of the body that are necessary to communicate effectively with others about aspects of cumulative trauma. Some of the most commonly used terms are provided in the attached glossary. Illustrations are also provided in Figures A1 and A2.

Glossary

Abduction/Adduction

Abduction	— movement away from the central axis of the body — away from the median plane.
Adduction	— movement toward the central axis of the body — toward the median plane.
Deviation	— a change or alteration, as in the following:
Radial deviation	— bending the hand at the wrist in the direction of the thumb.
Ulnar deviation	— bending the hand at the wrist in the direction of the little finger.

Flexion/Extension

Flexion	— movement that decreases the angle between two adjacent bones.
Extension	— movement that increases the angle between two adjacent bones.

Pronation/Supination

Pronation	— medial rotation of the forearm that brings the palm of the hand downward (turning the wrist so as to have the palm down).
Supination	— lateral rotation of the forearm that brings the palm of the hand upward (turning the wrist so as to have the palm up).

Lateral/Medial

Lateral   — structures farther to the sides, away from
                         the midline.
Medial   — structures of the body nearest the midline.

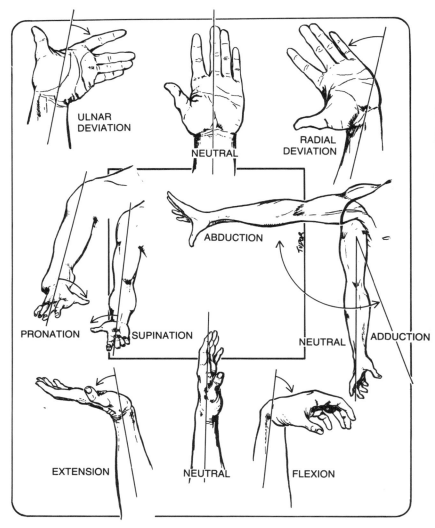

Figure A1.   Positions of the hand and arm.

Planes (see Figure A2)

Coronal plane   — a vertical plane perpendicular to the
                         median plane that divides the body into
                         anterior (front) and posterior (back)
                         segments.
Frontal plane   — another name for coronal plane.
Sagittal plane   — the median plane (called midsagittal) or
                         any plane parallel to it that divides the body
                         into right and left parts.
Transverse plane —   a plane at right angles to both the sagittal
                         and coronal planes dividing the body into
                         superior and inferior portions.

Effort

Dynamic effort — rhythmic alteration of contraction and extension, tension and relaxation.

Static effort — prolonged state of muscle contraction. Muscles remain in a state of heightened tension; blood is not flowing through the muscle, and no useful work is visible.

Static work — work that occurs when effort must be made to hold the body in a certain position instead of directing that effort to a task such as grasping.

Forces

External forces — forces applied to the body by outside objects (e.g., weight of a box being held or carried).

Internal forces — those forces generated by the muscles as a result of muscle tendon action (e.g., holding or carrying a weight).

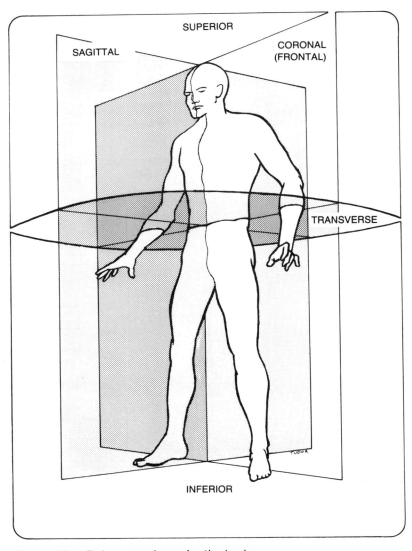

Figure A2. Reference planes for the body.

Appendix B

Medical Diagnosis and Treatment[a]

This section illustrates how the diagnostic process works and identifies some of the general procedures used by the medical profession in treating these disorders. Additional information dealing with medical diagnosis and treatment of musculoskeletal injuries can be found by consulting the reference sources listed at the end of this chapter.

How and why diagnoses are made

Determining the cause and the type of a CTD is important for several reasons. First, a correct diagnosis is needed to select the most useful or effective medical treatment. Second, the cause of a CTD must be identified so that the stressful activity can be avoided. If the stressful activity cannot be avoided, then the activity or job must be modified in some way so as to reduce or eliminate trauma to the body. Third, a diagnosis lets the patient know what to expect, since the usual courses of common CTDs are known. For example, many shoulder problems eventually result in chronic pain with any large movement of the shoulder joint. Such news is understandably distressing to the patient. However, once the diagnosis is correctly established, the patient can be reassured that the pain will gradually disappear over a 6-month to 1-year period with some form of physical rehabilitation and with avoidance of certain shoulder movements. Finally, a specific diagnosis is usually necessary to establish the work-related nature of a CTD. If the CTD is correctly diagnosed as work-related, the patient is usually eligible for compensation for the cost of medical treatment and lost time that may not otherwise be available.

The diagnosis of a particular problem should contain several parts. First, the specific part of the body affected should be identified. For example, the cause of pain and tingling in the fourth and fifth fingers could be pressure on the ulnar nerve at the elbow. Such symptoms might occur with work requiring elbows to rest on a work bench for long periods.

The second part of the diagnosis is to describe the degree of impairment or the extent of the loss of function. For example, in

---

[a]Prepared by L. Fine, M.D.

tendinitis of the shoulder, the ability of the patient to raise his or her arm should be evaluated. There are standard methods for medical professionals to precisely assess and record the degree of impairment.

The third component of a diagnosis is to determine what, if anything, triggered the sudden onset of the symptoms and what the underlying long-term cause is. Often, changes in recent work or leisure-time activities may trigger some pain in a joint or a muscle that was injured or weakened by events that occurred many years earlier.

History — The patient's experience

The first and most important information used in making a diagnosis is the patient's description of what bothers him or her, how the problem started, how it has progressed, and what makes it better or worse. This history can be useful in several ways.

The first use of the history is to help determine the severity of the problem through the patient's own assessment. For example, a victim of carpal tunnel syndrome may notice that grasping motions with his or her thumb are becoming progressively weaker. This observation may indicate a serious abnormality in the median nerve function and a wasting away of the muscles that move the thumb. A history of increasing difficulty with opening jars or dropping of tools is evidence that the carpal tunnel syndrome is severe.

The second use for the history is to help the examiner determine whether the problem is a nerve or a tendon disorder. In nerve disorders, cramping pain or numbness and tingling are often reported. The sensation is often compared with the familiar "pins and needles" feeling that occurs when the hand "falls asleep". Tendon problems usually result in dull, aching pain that is often worse in the evening. Also, the patient will usually limit the motion of the affected tendon. For example, patients with shoulder problems often stop combing their hair or reaching into their back pocket with the affected arm. Though symptoms sometimes suggest which tissue has been injured or damaged, they are often not very specific. Discomfort that wakes the patient from sleep occurs both with carpal tunnel syndrome and tendinitis of the shoulder.

The third way that the history can be useful is in helping to locate the site of the problem. For example, numbness in the hand and fingers is common to both thoracic outlet and carpal tunnel syndrome. But the numbess is most commonly felt in the fourth and fifth fingers for thoracic outlet syndrome, and in the first three fingers for carpal tunnel syndrome.

Occasionally, referred pain (that which is felt in a body part far removed from the site where it actually originates) can be confused with pain from a joint or tendon. The source of referred pain is often an internal organ and may represent a serious medical problem. For example, gall bladder problems often cause shoulder pain.

The physical examination

The physical examination for a CTD involves several components. The first is called **inspection**, and it simply involves observing the patient. The examiner looks for asymmetry between the two sides of the body or for other visible irregularities like a ganglion or swelling.

The second part of the examination is called **range of motion maneuvers (ROM)**. These include active and passive, and resisted motions.[1] In passive ROMs, the patient allows the examiner to move the arm through a set of positions. This procedure is especially useful for determining whether a problem within a joint is present. When a joint is moved by the examiner, the muscles and tendons surrounding the joint are generally relaxed. The major stress is usually located **within the joint**, so if pain is caused by the motion, a joint problem is suspected.

Resisted ROMs test the muscle tendon structures. The patient attempts to move his or her arm while the examiner holds the arm steady. As a result, the muscles are contracted and tendons pulled without joint motion. Thus, the resisted motions are a better test of tendon and muscle function than of joint motion. If the resisted motions are more painful than the appropriate passive motions, the problem often involves a tendon.

In active ROM tests, the patient moves his arms by himself. These tests combine the testing of both tendons and joint structures. They are a good screening test for a particular joint. For example, if one can perform the three simple motions illustrated in Figure B1, then it is unlikely that a serious CTD exists in the muscles or tendons of the shoulder joint. Subtle signs can be observed during these motions which indicate a serious problem.

In the third part of the physical examination, the examiner presses with his or her fingers against a part of the body to determine whether there are areas of tenderness. This is called **palpation**. This procedure can be very useful in discovering the particular source of the problem. For example, palpation is used to locate which of the shoulder tendons is the most inflamed. Since palpation can cause generalized pain that could lead to misleading symptoms, it would normally be performed after ROM testing.

The fourth part of the physical examination tests arterial blood vessels and peripheral nerves of the upper extremities. In thoracic outlet syndrome, for example, the pulse at the wrist may be noticeably weaker when the patient raises the affected arm straight up and turns his or her head to the side. This procedure is known as the Adson maneuver.

Laboratory tests

Laboratory and specialized electronic tests may be performed after the physical examination. For example, if the patient reports loss of sensation and control of the hand, a carpal tunnel

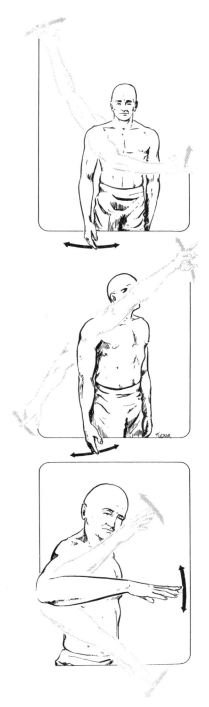

Figure B1. Motions for determining CTDs of the shoulder.

syndrome (CTS) condition may be suspected. A special electrodiagnostic test is available that is capable of determining if the ulnar and median nerves in the hand have been damaged. A key diagnostic condition of CTS is entrapment and injury of the median nerve inside the carpal tunnel of the wrist. When a nerve has been damaged, the velocity of the nerve impulses are reduced. By measuring the velocity of the median nerve and comparing it to the velocity of the ulnar nerve a more rigorous diagnosis can often be made. As with many electrodiagnostic techniques, however, the procedure is very sensitive to artifacts, such as electrode placement, temperature, and accurate calibration. Electromyographic (EMG) diagnostic techniques have also been used to assess muscle activity. The majority of CTDs, however, seldom require such elaborate methods for diagnosis if a thorough physical examination has been conducted.

As an alternative to X-rays and dye-induced arthrograms, a new technique called magnetic resonance imaging (MRI) is being used to provide images of soft tissue, which includes tendons, ligaments and muscles. MRI relies on the interaction between the body's normally aligned hydrogen protons and radio frequency waves to produce a computerized image of an intact structure or a joint. By improving the diagnostic information, MRI should reduce the incidence of unneeded surgery.

The assessment

The final stage of the diagnostic process is the assessment. The examiner attempts to review the mass of information collected, synthesizes it into an overall analysis of the problem, and decides on the proper course of treatment.

The successful treatment of CTDs depends on an accurate diagnosis that provides the following information:

(1) A precise anatomical location of the disorder. This step is important, because some treatments, such as drug injections into an inflamed tendon, require accurate contact with the injured body part.
(2) Characterization of the extent of damage. More severe injuries may require prompt surgical repair. In carpal tunnel syndrome, for example, it is generally agreed that surgery should be seriously considered once the patient shows signs of weakness and wasting away of the muscles at the base of the thumb.
(3) Determination of whether the disorder is a cumulative trauma or some other condition. The information from the exam is reviewed to see if it fits the pattern of one or more CTDs. Often a list is made of the most likely possibilities, including non-CTD problems such as an infected joint or arthritis. Pinpointing the basic type of disorder is the single most influential factor in selecting an appropriate treatment.
(4) Determination of the duration of the CTD and its response to previous treatments. Failure of previous therapy to

relieve a CTD may indicate that the previous diagnosis
was wrong or that the patient is still performing an activity
at home or work that is reinjuring the damaged body part.

Medical treatment

This section presents some of the general principles that
guide the treatment of CTDs. These principles are not presented
in sufficient detail to be of use in prescribing treatment; rather
they give the interested reader a basic understanding of the
general treatment process. The intention is to provide sufficient
information to facilitate intelligent discussions between doctors
and patients and other concerned parties about the treatment of
CTDs.

The patient is generally interested in several goals:

(1) To be able to live and continue working without significant
pain.
(2) To have a treatment plan that will minimize side effects,
involve the least disruption to one's life, and not be too
costly.
(3) To have a treatment plan that will restore him or her to a
healthy state in the shortest possible time.

Often trade-offs are involved in choosing a particular type of
treatment. The doctor and patient must discuss the possible
choices and the patient's priorities and preferences. Jointly they
should establish a set of goals and a time frame for
accomplishing them.

Non-medical people and patients often fail to understand or
accept readily the fact that weeks or often months may be
required for medical therapy to be successful. The major goal of
therapy is to eliminate or at least sharply reduce the physical
stresses that caused or aggravated the CTD. Once this stress
has been eliminated, the body's natural repair process can take
place. Recovery often requires a long period during which work
activities must be restricted.

If the recovery period is long, or if the preliminary treatment
fails, difficulties for the patients and their families can be very
troublesome. But it is important not to take a short-term view of a
chronic illness. The "quack" doctor will intentionally attempt to
provide immediate and temporary relief at the expense of a long-
term cure. With CTDs, the illusory quick cure may lead only to
future problems. What is required is a long-term strategy that is
shared and negotiated with the patient. This strategy must be
flexible, and it requires modification during the treatment
process.

Treatment strategies

A treatment strategy usually tries the simplest approaches
first. They should be the least costly and the least painful, and
they should have the fewest side effects. These approaches are
called **conservative treatments**. If this approach fails, the doctor
may try more elaborate treatments such as the use of special
drugs or even surgery in extreme cases.

Conservative treatment of CTDs combines four types of therapies:

(1) Restricting motion and splinting.
(2) Applying heat or cold.
(3) Medications and injections.
(4) Special exercise.

Restricting motion

The first major type of therapy is to avoid the activities that cause pain or stress the injured body area. This often entails the use of work restrictions. A splint may also be used to immobilize movement of the joint or muscles. The aim is to reduce pain or inflammation by supporting the body part in a position of low stress.

In the case of carpal tunnel syndrome, for example, the following treatments may be used: If the condition has not been present for more than a year and if there is no evidence of muscle deterioration and weakness, a simple, very lightweight splint can be molded for the patient's wrist. The splint illustrated in Figure B2 maintains the wrist in a slight extension yet permits and assists finger and thumb movement. Patients are instructed to avoid extensive wrist motion, particularly when pinching or grasping.

Splinting and taking aspirin or other mild analgesics usually provide significant alleviation of symptoms. This method may require months of persistence, but it is often successful. If there is significant muscle deterioration and chronic pain, a more radical form of treatment may be required.

Splints for immobilization of a painful joint can lead to three types of problems. The first is that the inactivity can weaken muscle. The problem, however, is not major because loss of muscle tone is reversible after treatment ends. The second problem is that long periods of inactivity (4 weeks or more) can cause loss of normal range of motion in the splinted joints. This is a particular problem with the shoulder if it is immobilized. The third problem is that if a worker with a splint is assigned jobs that require major movements of the splinted area, these motions may be even more stressful with the splint than without it. A transfer to a different job needs to be considered.

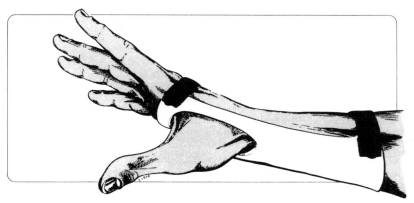

Figure B2.   Splint for carpal tunnel syndrome.

Heat and cold

The second major type of therapy is the application of heat or cold to relieve pain and perhaps facilitate the repair process. Definite evidence exists to support the usefulness of heat or cold for temporary pain relief, especially before periods of physical therapy. Much less evidence supports a major role for such application in speeding the healing process.

Therapeutic heating can be subdivided into two categories: superficial heating (such as the use of a heating pad, hot packs or a sauna) and diathermy, or deep heating (shortwave and ultrasound). The type of heating used depends on the location of the injury. Ultrasound may be used on a deep muscle injury and a heat lamp on an injury closer to the skin's surface. Heat increases the blood circulation in muscles and tendons that are close to the skin's surface.

Heat may be recommended for pain relief for minor strains where there is no swelling. Where there is an injury that is causing significant inflammation, however, the application of heat should be avoided for at least 48 hours. Heat will increase the flow of blood to the injured area, causing increased internal bleeding and swelling. After 48 hours heat may be applied to temporarily ease the discomfort of sore and tense muscles. For the majority of CTDs, however, there is no evidence that heat by itself can help heal painful scar tissue, reduce inflammation and swelling, or relieve pressure on a nerve.

Ice, if applied immediately after an injury or overuse strain, promotes recovery by reducing pain and swelling, which allows more mobility. For strains and sprains active movement is beneficial. For CTDs some movement may also be beneficial, but vigorous movements or exercising the hand or arm may further aggravate the condition. Ice is clearly inappropriate for Raynaud's disease (vibration syndrome), rheumatoid arthritis and diabetic conditions.

Medication

The third major type of therapy is the use of medication to reduce inflammation and pain. Three types of drugs are used for treating CTDs: aspirin, non-steroidal anti-inflammatory drugs and injected corticosteroids.

All of these drugs are effective in reducing inflammation. Inflammation is a natural response of the body to injury or physical stress. The repair processes of the body can often repair the damage completely if the inflammation is stopped soon enough. However, it can be dangerous to disrupt the body's ability to initiate an inflammatory response, since it is an important defense against infections, and has many other useful purposes.

Aspirin is probably the most commonly used drug for CTDs, and it has two useful actions: relieving pain and reducing the inflammatory response. The dose of aspirin needed to reduce inflammation is higher than the amount needed to relieve pain. Though aspirin is a safe drug, there are side effects, which include heartburn, nausea and gastrointestinal problems. Risks of developing problems can be reduced if aspirin is taken with liquid or food

More than 25 drugs are categorized as **non-steroidal anti-inflammatory drugs (NSAID)**. The actions of these drugs are believed to be similar to aspirin. They differ in that most are much more expensive, and some are much longer-acting than aspirin and may be given once a day. Experts differ as to whether these drugs are a major advance over aspirin. Most believe that some of the NSAIDs are less likely to cause gastrointestinal symptoms than aspirin, but evidence is less convincing that the risks of serious ulcer or bleeding problems are reduced.

Injections of **corticosteroids** (such as cortisone) into the inflamed site in the case of tendinitis or bursitis can often provide effective relief, but may also impede the healing process. These injections have been used in the past with varying degrees of success for a large number of CTDs. As long as injections are not used frequently, their main risks are infections (which is very unusual) and rupture of a tendon (if repeated large volumes of medicine are used). Injections can frequently cause a temporary increase in pain for 24 to 48 hours.

All of the drugs discussed so far are best viewed as secondary forms of treatment to make the patient more comfortable. Work restriction and splinting may also be used to allow recovery. Prevention, however, should be aimed at reducing the levels of physical stress through job redesign.

Stretching and exercise

Stretching is an important link between sedentary activities and work. Stretching promotes circulation, increases the range of motion, and reduces muscle tension. Stretching, if done properly, will also prevent injuries such as muscle strains. Though stretching is routinely recommended for prevention of low back problems, there is also a need to stretch the upper body prior to work. Stretching prescriptions have been devised for almost every type of activity and part of the body.

Various forms of exercise can be used to maintain or restore strength to an injured joint and its surrounding tendon–muscle units. With respect to CTDs, exercise is probably most important in the case of shoulder disorders. For hand or wrist disorders exercise should be avoided since it will likely aggravate the existing condition. For people with CTDs, a physical therapist should be consulted before any type of stretching or exercise program is initiated.

Conclusions about treatments

One of the most important aspects of any treatment program is to ensure cooperation between the patient and others (employer, supervisor and family members) who can have a major impact on the patient's level of exposure and general well-being. Thus, the patient and doctor must communicate sufficiently to ensure that the patient understands the causes of the injury, the likely course of treatment and the overall outcome.

If a doctor recommends a non-conservative treatment such as surgery or drugs that may have serious side effects, then it is even more important that the patient understands the reasons for such treatment, its risk, and the expected outcome.

Finally, if a complete and permanent recovery is expected, it is important that **the worker is not returned to the same job or task that precipitated the CTD**. This may require establishing a communication network that includes the patient's physician, a top management person, a person from the company's loss control department, the worker's supervisor, key health and safety staff and worker representatives. Ultimately, a successful program for the treatment, control and prevention of CTDs depends on a team approach where open dialogue is encouraged and rewarded.

Suggested reading

Anderson, B.A., 1980, *Stretching*. (Bolinas, CA: Shelter Publications).

Benjamin, B.E., 1984, *Listen to Your Pain*. (London: Penguin Books). Useful as a layman's resource for identifying bursitis and muscle and tendon injuries.

Birnbaum, J.S., 1982, *The Musculoskeletal Manual*. (New York: Academic Press). A practical illustrated guide to the diagnosis and treatment of a wide range of musculoskeletal injuries, including most of the CTDs.

Cailliet, R., 1983, *Soft Tissue Pain and Disability*. (Philadelphia: F.A. Davis Company).

Other valuable books by Dr. Cailliet include *Shoulder Pain, Hand Pain and Impairment* and *Neck and Arm Pain*.

Appendix C

CTD Statistics: Prevalence, Incidence and Severity[b]

Any system that is used to measure the frequency of occupational CTDs should have the following attributes:

(1) The system should indicate the rate at which the disorders occur in a specified group of workers.
(2) The system should be able to compare the rates of disorders between two groups of workers.
(3) The system should be able to identify areas (e.g., plants, departments, sections, job titles) in which CTDs are emerging or unacceptably high.
(4) The system should be able to measure progress (or lack of it) in efforts to control disorders.

Three pieces of information are needed to compute a meaningful frequency rate: the numerator of the fraction (the number of workers in a specified group that experience a disorder), the denominator of the fraction (the total number of workers in the specified group), and the period of time in which the disorders occurred.[2]

Prevalence and incidence are often used to measure the frequency of a disease or disorder. Simply defined, **prevalence** is a dimension-less unit that gives the frequency of a disorder, or the proportion of a population that experiences it, at a specified point in time. The following case is an example:

A plant that manufactures computer circuit boards employed 135 assembly line workers on July 1, 1983. On that date, all of these workers were given a physical examination to detect cases of carpal tunnel syndrome. Five cases were found during the examinations. The prevalence rate for this population was therefore computed as 5/135, or 0.037.

The **incidence** of a disorder is the number of new cases that come into being during a specific period of time. For occupational disorders, time is usually measured in terms of exposure hours to a job, in addition to calendar time.

The **incidence rate** is the number of new cases in a population per specified unit of exposure time. Before the passage of the U.S. Occupational Safety and Health Act (OSHA Act) in 1970,

---

[b]Section prepared by W. M. Keyserling.

most industries computed incidence rates as the number of cases of a disorder per million hours of exposure (ANSI, 1969). Since the implementation of the Act, most industries have adopted the OSHA procedure that uses 200,000 hours as the standard unit of exposure time. The following example illustrates the OSHA method:

> In the previous example, the circuit board manufacturer employed an average of 128 full-time employees during calendar year 1982. (A full-time employee works 40 hours per week, 50 weeks per year for an exposure time of 2000 hours per year.) During that year, six new cases of carpal tunnel syndrome (CTS) were diagnosed among assembly line workers. The OSHA-computed incidence rate of CTS for the year can be computed using the formula:[3]

$$\text{Incidence rate} = \frac{\text{Cases} \times 200,000}{\text{Hours worked}} = \frac{6 \times 200,000}{128 \times 2,000} = 4 \cdot 69$$

Substituting plant data into the equation, the incidence rate of CTS was found to be 4·69 during 1983. This may be considered a moderate incidence level, and may serve as an early indicator of an emerging problem. An ergonomic hazard analysis should be conducted to determine if the incidence rate represents a trend requiring some immediate intervention or only a temporary condition that is self-limiting.

Severity statistics attempt to describe the seriousness of a disorder in terms of its cost to an employer. Severity is not a measure of disease frequency. A commonly used measure is the **American National Standards Institute (ANSI) Severity Rate**, defined as the number of work days lost during a calendar year per million hours of work time.[4] Other commonly used severity measures include:

(1) Number of days lost per employee per year or number of days lost per 100 employees per year.
(2) Worker's compensation cost per employee per year or per 100 employees per year.
(3) Number of days lost per case of a given type of disorder or injury.
(4) Worker's compensation cost per case of a given type of disorder or injury.

Because of the lack of standardization in severity statistics, it is often impossible to compare the experience of one plant with that of another.

Advantages and limitations of statistical measures

None of the statistics discussed above is the best single measure for describing CTDs. The primary advantage of **prevalence** statistics is that they describe the proportion of a population affected by a disorder at an instant in time. This information may be helpful in identifying problem jobs where CTDs are unacceptably high. However, because prevalence rates are computed for a given point in time, repeated observations should be made to assure the stability of the statistics.

The major problem with prevalence measures is that they depend on two factors; the development of new cases of a disorder and the duration of a case once it develops. To identify causal factors that explain the occurrence of a disorder, **incidence** statistics are preferable to prevalence statistics.

By plotting incidence rates over time, it is possible to determine changes in the rate of new cases. If there is a sudden increase in the incidence rate, one can attempt to identify the cause (e.g., a change in production methods that was implemented before the increase). Analysis of incidence rates is also useful in evaluating the effectiveness of programs that are implemented to control CTDs.

The principle use of **severity** statistics is to determine the costs associated with repetitive trauma disorders. These statistics can be plotted over time to assess the costs of the problem and the effectiveness of control programs. A potential weakness of severity statistics is that they are affected by many factors associated with the recovery from a disorder (e.g., quality and timeliness of medical treatment, success of rehabilitation programs, and the ability to find gainful employment for a worker recovering from a CTD).

Information provided by severity statistics can be very useful in evaluating the effectiveness of medical services and rehabilitation programs. However, these statistics provide almost no information regarding the causes of disorders, and they are of limited use in developing prevention programs.

In summary, several statistics are available for describing the frequency and costs associated with CTDs. Since each statistic has certain limitations, it is desirable to use several types of statistics to describe and evaluate the problem.

Response measures for evaluating CTDs

The frequency measures discussed in the above section are highly sensitive to the procedures and criteria that are used to classify and count occupational CTDs. These issues are discussed below.

Cumulative trauma disorders are different from most occupational injuries in that they do not result from a clearly defined event or accident. Instead, the disorder may gradually develop over an extended period. When an employee recognizes symptoms of the disorder, it is often difficult to identify a specific occupational cause, since there is no associated mishap or accident to flag the occasion. In some instances, the early symptoms of a disorder may not occur while a worker is performing his or her job, and they may not be associated with work activities. An example of this phenomenon is the nocturnal paresthesia often experienced in the early stages of carpal tunnel syndrome. It may not be obvious to the patient that the feelings of pain, tingling or numbness that occur at night are caused by repetitive hand and wrist activities that occur during the day.

Counting systems based on identification of symptoms

Conventional systems for recording occupational injuries and illnesses usually require the condition to be clearly related to an occupational activity or event for the case to be recorded (ANSI, 1969). As a result, these systems tend to under-report CTDs when a specific cause cannot be identified.

An alternative method is to count all cases of CTD, even if occupational activities are only partially or potentially responsible for the case. Such a system is based on identifying symptoms of CTD instead of specific causes. An attractive feature of identifying symptoms is that this method recognizes that CTDs can be caused by normal work activities instead of deviations from the normal (i.e., accidents). If this approach is accepted, then appropriate investigative procedures can be used for identifying the CTD causes (e.g., tool and equipment design, work methods, etc.). Obviously, this approach generates higher frequency statistics than the conventional method for counting cases.

Counting systems based on the severity of the disorder

Frequency statistics also depend on the type of response measure used to count cases of CTDs. If the counting system recognizes only lost-time cases or Workers' compensation cases, relatively low prevalence and incidence rates will be computed because the counting system recognizes only those cases that have progressed to the point at which a person can no longer work at any job.

A system of counting based on severity also misses those cases in which an employer transfers the affected worker to another job that has fewer stresses that could either cause or aggravate the disorder. The principle advantage of a counting system that measures lost-time is that it recognizes only the most severe CTD cases. A main disadvantage of a system based on severity is that it ignores CTDs in the early stages. In other words, by the time CTDs are recognized as an important problem at a worksite, some of the workers with CTDs may have progressed to the point where substantial costs (in terms of lost time and Workers' compensation payments) are incurred. Hence, the main disadvantage of a prevalence rate based on severity is that it may be insensitive to early indicators of CTDs, and may under-estimate the overall significance of CTD problems at a workplace.

If the scope of the counting system is expanded to include all OSHA recordable cases, any employee complaint requiring medical attention (other than first aid) would be counted. This system would be more sensitive to early signs of CTDs than the system discussed above. Naturally, it would result in higher frequency rates.

Counting systems that are based on either lost-time cases or OSHA recordable cases usually include only those situations in which an employee takes the initiative to seek medical treatment from his own physician or from the employer's medical service. Moreover, if the worker seeks private treatment, he or she will usually have to report this to the company's personnel or medical department. In addition, a copy of the physician's diagnosis will be needed to support the work-related nature of the disorder. Hence, unless the worker takes the initiative to obtain medical treatment for the CTD, and reports the disorder to the proper office in the company, the case will never be recorded. The only way to count such cases is to survey the workforce for symptoms and complaints of CTDs.

Counting systems based on employee surveys

The principle advantage of counting systems based on employee surveys is that they are more sensitive to CTDs in their earliest stages of development. This information may be very useful in the development of programs to control stresses that cause the disorders before they progress to serious stages. A disadvantage of this type of counting system is that it over-counts cases, since some CTD symptoms result from non-occupational causes and surveyed employees might report non-existent symptoms. Not surprisingly, this type of counting system generates the highest frequency statistics of the methods discussed.

Counting systems based on occupational injury statistics

Standardized practices that are currently in use for recording occupational injury data (e.g., the U.S. Bureau of Labor Statistics, Supplementary Data System, SDS) were originally designed for recording information pertaining to work accidents.* Because CTDs typically cannot be associated with a clearly defined event or accident, the recording systems are not well suited for collecting information on these injuries. In fact, no methods are presently available for using existing data bases to accurately estimate the frequency of CTDs and their cost on a national level.

Despite these problems, NIOSH completed a study to assess the magnitude and distribution of wrist disorders that are caused by repetitive motions and exertions.[5] In this study, workers' compensation data for the calendar year 1979 were obtained from the 30 states that participate in the SDS. To be included in the analysis, the compensation claim associated with the case had to satisfy three criteria:

(1) The **nature of the injury** had to be either inflammation of musculo-skeletal tissue (e.g., joints, tendons, muscles) or peripheral nerves.
(2) The **body part affected** had to be the wrist.
(3) The **cause or onset** of the disorder could *not* have been mechanical impact. Instead, the disorder must have been caused by repetitive motion or pressure, or by overexertion.

---

*The SDS was designed to standardize occupational injury and illness data from State Workers' compensation systems to achieve some degree of national comparability. The source of information for SDS is the reports of injury and illness which employers and insurance carriers submit to State Worker's Compensation Offices.

During 1979, a total of 58,698 workers' compensation claims were filed for wrist injuries in the 30 states that reported to the SDS. Approximately 6 per cent of these claims were classified as cumulative trauma injuries using the criteria listed above. The average cost to settle a CTD claim was $1498.[5]

Incident ratios were computed for wrist injuries in seven different industry groups (Table C1). (Note: **Incident ratio** was defined as the number of claims per 100,000 workers. The denominators of the ratios in Table C1 were estimated using census data. Exposure hours were not available; therefore incidence rates could not be computed.) Manufacturing operations had the highest incident ratio of all industry groups, with 20·1 wrist injuries per 100,000 workers. Incident ratios were also computed on the basis of occupation. The 12 occupations with the highest incident ratios are presented in Table C2. Based on the reported claims butchers experienced the highest rate of CTDs.[5]

Table C1.   Industry-specific ratios of 1979 non-impact wrist compensation claims for 30 states.

Manufacturing	20·1
Construction	9·1
Trade	3·7
Services	2·4
Mining	2·4
Transportation	2·2
Finance	0·9
Total	8·3

Table C2.   Incident ratio of 1979 non-impact wrist disorder claims in 30 states by occupational title.

Occupation	Claims per 100,000 workers
Butchers	222·1
Miscellaneous laborers	141·5
Assemblers	133·7
Fishermen, oystermen	94·0
Bottling, canning operatives	89·3
Polishers/buffers/sanders	57·3
Shoemakers	54·2
Punch press operators	44·9
Sawyers	44·7
Miscellaneous operatives	43·0
Material handlers	42·2
Packers	40·2

The statistics developed in the NIOSH study do not fully describe the magnitude of the CTD problem in the U.S. for the following reasons:

(1) The study, described above, was limited to disorders of the wrist. As discussed elsewhere in this manual, the shoulders, elbows, hands and fingers are also common sites of cumulative trauma complaints.

(2) The study was limited to CTD cases that resulted in the filing (and eventual settlement) of a workers' compensation claim. To qualify for compensation, the injured worker must have missed a specified minimum number of work days (typically ranging from 3 to 7 days, depending on the laws of the state where the claim was filed). Lost workday cases that did not exceed the minimum were not counted. Cases where an injured worker was assigned to an alternative job were not counted. Cases in which a worker continued to work while injured were not counted.

(3) Because the relationship between work activities and the development of CTD was not always obvious, some

workers who experienced CTDs may not have filed workers' compensation claims. (In situations where a worker was adequately covered by private or even company health and disability insurance, there would have been no reason to file for compensation.)

(4) Considerable differences exist among the states in the definition and recognition of CTD from the standpoint of compensation.

(5) Not all workers in the U.S. are covered by the workers' compensation system.

Case studies of CTD costs and frequency

Because of the problems discussed here, it has been difficult to estimate accurately the magnitude or cost of CTD in the United States. However, several studies have recently been performed to measure the frequency and/or cost of CTDs within specific populations. The results of selected studies are summarized in the cases presented in the following subsections:

Case 1: Electronic parts manufacturer

Plant A is a medium-sized facility that manufactures small electronic parts for circuit boards and other electronic equipment. Depending on the demand for the products produced, hourly employment ranges between 800 and 1000. Most of the workers are women aged 20 to 40 who live in the rural communities near the plant. Virtually all of the production jobs in the plant are sedentary and consist of repetitive hand tasks (e.g., loading and unloading parts to racks, jigs, fixtures and machines; operating machine tools, using hand tools such as wire cutters, and inspecting). These jobs are performed while standing or sitting at a workbench. Most employees are paid under an incentive system that awards bonuses for each unit processed above a base rate.

Management became concerned about CTDs (particularly carpal tunnel syndrome) in the plant when the medical department reported an increase in lost-time cases. A study was initiated to determine the cost of these problems. In this study, workers' compensation claims were reviewed to identify cases of CTDs that resulted in a compensation payment. During the 6-month period in which claims were reviewed, six carpal tunnel claims were settled. With the procedures developed in the NIOSH study discussed above, this figure converts to an incident ratio of more than 1300 cases per 100,000 workers per year. Table C2 compares this rate with wrist disorders in other occupational groups. The sum of medical costs (surgical fees, hospital fees, occupational therapy, etc.) and disability payments averaged approximately $2400 per case. There was, however, a wide range in the cost of settlements, from a low of about $200 to a high of more than $8000. Furthermore, the typical case resulted in about 7 weeks of lost time.

Although the above numbers seem high, they underestimate the severity of CTDs in the plant. First, they were limited to counting only those cases of carpal tunnel syndrome that resulted in a compensation claim. Less severe cases of carpal tunnel syndrome and cases of other CTDs were not counted. Second, they were limited to cases in which final settlement was reached during the 6-month period of the study. Several additional carpal tunnel cases occurred, but were not settled during the period covered by the study.

Case 2: Metal fabrication

Plant B manufactures air filters for a variety of engines and office machines. The hourly workforce fluctuates between about 50 and 100, depending on the sales of the plant's products. Production jobs in the plant occur in two major areas — metal fabricating and product assembly. In the metal fabricating area (about 15 percent of the hourly workforce) employees operate stamping presses, press brakes, and manipulate machine tools to form the metal frames that house the filters. In the assembly area (about 75 percent of the workforce) employees cut and break paper filter elements, install the elements into the metal housing assembly, and clean the final assembly using putty knives and other hand tools. Virtually all of the jobs in the metal fabricating and assembly areas involve repetitive exertions of the hands and upper extremities. The balance of the hourly workforce (about 10 percent) performs miscellaneous activities such as maintenance or shipping and receiving.

In 1981, NIOSH performed a health hazard evaluation at the plant after receiving a request from the employees' union. At the time of the NIOSH visit, 96 hourly workers were employed. A review of medical and insurance records revealed that 15 of these workers were initially diagnosed as having carpal tunnel syndrome while working at the plant. Of these, 11 had undergone surgery to decompress the median nerve in the affected hand(s). While at the plant, NIOSH medical personnel distributed questionnaires and performed physical evaluations on the 96 employees. As a result of these procedures, 16 additional "suspected" cases of carpal tunnel syndrome were discovered. (A case was classified as suspected if the worker experienced symptoms consistent with the carpal tunnel syndrome.)

Counting only the 15 confirmed cases (those with a positive diagnosis of carpal tunnel syndrome before the NIOSH visit) and using payroll records, the incidence rate was found to be 7·5 cases per 200,000 hours. The corresponding prevalence rate based on confirmed cases was computed as 0·16. By adding the suspected cases, the prevalence rate increased to 0·32 for the plant.

The above discussion of prevalence rates shows how any statistic of disease frequency is largely dependent on the criteria that are used to define a case. By relaxing the definition from "confirmed diagnosis" to "symptoms consistent with carpal tunnel syndrome", the prevalence rate virtually doubled.

Case 3: Poultry processing plant

In Plant C, turkey carcasses travel down an overhead conveyor belt and are disassembled into a variety of poultry products. Many of the jobs on the conveyor line require repetitive hand motions to cut and separate parts of the carcass.[6]

By reviewing injury logs that covered an 8-month period, the morbidity patterns for CTDs in Plant C were identified. Disorders of the hand, wrist, forearm and elbow were classified into one of the following categories:

Nervous – A diagnosed injury or illness of a nerve, or numbness in the upper extremity that could not be attributed to an acute episode.

Tendinous – An inflammation, tearing, or any other injury or illness of a tendon or tendon sheath that could not be attributed to an acute episode.

Non-specific – Any complaint (e.g., soreness, aching, swelling) that could not be attributed to an acute episode.

Incidence rates (per 200,000 hours) were computed in Table C3 for each of the three categories of disorders for eight different areas of the plant.[6]

Table C3.   *Analysis of frequencies and incidence rates of CTDs by area in a poultry products plant.*

Department	Hours	Nervous		Tendinous		Non-specific		Total	
		No.	I.R.	No.	I.R.	No.	I.R.	No.	I.R.
Trimming	58,092	0	0·0	0	0·0	6	20·7	6	20·7
Boning	114,794	1	1·7	1	1·7	8	13·9	10	17·4
Skinning	15,438	0	0·0	1	13·0	9	116·9	10	129·6
Parts	52,262	0	0·0	0	0·0	1	6·2	1	6·2
Pan roast	30,400	1	6·6	0	0·0	1	6·6	2	13·2
Curing	5,024	0	0·0	0	0·0	1	39·8	1	39·8
Cook roll	11,538	0	0·0	1	17·3	0	0·0	1	17·3
Sanitation	13,310	0	0·0	0	0·0	1	7·4	1	7·4
Total	501,668	2	0·8	3	1·2	27	10·8	32	12·8

No. = Number.
I.R. = Incidence.
Notes: Cases per 200,000 work hours.

Several important observations can be made from Table C3. Clearly, a relationship exists between the department and the incidence rate of CTDs. For example, the incidence rate in the (thigh) skinning department (129·6) was more than 20 times the rate in the (turkey) parts department (6·2). The relationships between work activities and CTDs are discussed elsewhere in this manual (Chapter 4). This case illustrates the value of systematically reviewing injury data to identify potential problem areas for CTDs in a plant.

Note also that the overall incidence rate in Plant C was more than twice the reported rate in Plant B (see Case 2). Though there are many possible explanations for this difference (including differences in work activities), Plant B counted only diagnosed cases of carpal tunnel syndrome, whereas Plant C counted any complaint symptoms associated with a variety of CTDs. The latter counting method was more sensitive and therefore resulted in a higher rate.

Case 4: Clothing makers

This case is based on a study of 190 garment workers employed in seven garment shops.[7] Four of the shops were quite small, employing fewer than 15 production workers. Two of the shops employed more than 50 production workers.

Approximately two-thirds (125 of 190) of the study population were stitchers (i.e., sewing machine operators). This job involved rapid, repetitive hand motions to guide the fabric through the sewing machine. In addition, it was frequently necessary to hold the hands and wrists in awkward postures. All of the stitchers were females.

Seventeen workers (2 males and 15 females) were employed as pressers. This group operated utility steam pressing machines (similar to those that are found in most dry cleaning establishments). The job involved repetitive hand motions while placing garments on the pressing table, and repetitive shoulder actions while operating the machine.

Fifteen members of the study population (all females) were employed as floor help. This job involved carrying bundles of fabric between workstations, and it involved little, if any, repetitive hand work.

Eleven workers (8 males and 3 females) were employed as cutters. This job required the worker to operate an electric cutting machine to cut bulk fabric material into patterns. The job did not require repetitive hand motions, but it did require the operator to maintain the upper extremities in sustained and sometimes awkward postures.

The remainder of the population ($n = 22$) performed a variety of jobs. This group will be designated as "other" for the remainder of the discussion.

None of the seven shops was large enough to have an in-house medical clinic for treating work injuries or maintaining employee health records. As a result, it was impossible to review existing records to determine the existence of CTDs. To overcome this problem, a survey was conducted among the workers. The purpose of the survey was to determine the prevalence of symptoms (e.g., pain, numbness, tingling, swelling and stiffness) that could be related to disorders such as tendinitis, tenosynovitis, carpal tunnel syndrome, or degenerative joint disease. The results of this survey are presented in Table C4.

Table C4.   Prevalence of hand and wrist pain among garment industry workers.

Occupation	Number of workers	Subjects with pain	Prevalence rate
Stitchers	125	47	0·376
Pressers	17	5	0·294
Floor help	15	2	0·133
Cutter	11	3	0·273
Other	22	4	0·182
Total	190	61	0·321*

*Average.

The rate of hand and wrist pain among the surveyed workers was quite high. Almost one-third of the study population reported that they experienced persistent pain in their hands and wrists. The problem was greatest among the stitchers who reported a prevalence rate of 0·376. The problem was least among the floor help, who reported a prevalence rate of 0·133. In spite of the high prevalence rates, it is important to note that all of the participants in the study were performing their assigned jobs at the time of the study and therefore were not disabled by their pain. The reported pain, however, may have been a precursor to potentially disabling disorders and may have reduced productivity.

The prevalence rates reported in Case 4 were the highest of all the cases presented because pain was selected as a criterion for counting a case of CTD instead of the more stringent criteria used in the other cases. In addition, reports of pain were actively sought in Case 4 by surveying workers to identify cases of interest. In the other case studies, passive methods (e.g., review of workers' compensation records) were used to identify cases.

Identification of problem areas

Generating job-specific rates of CTD[c]

To determine whether a CTD problem exists on a given job or in a given area, it is necessary to collect the data required to compute job-specific or area-specific incidence rates.

Consider the information in Table C5 for hypothetical Plant Z. The plant employed an average of 1450 workers during 1981 in three different departments. A review of the OSHA log disclosed that there were 36 new cases of tendinitis in the plant during the year. According to payroll records, a total of 2·9 million hours were worked. Table C5 also gives the number of employees, tendinitis cases and work hours for each of the three departments.

Table C5. Tendinitis experience in hypothetical plant Z.

Item	Dept. A	Dept. B	Dept. C	Total Plant
Employees	450·0	300·0	700·0	1450·0
Hours worked*	900·0	600·0	1400·0	2900·0
Tendinitis cases	22·0	4·0	10·0	36·0
Incidence rate	4·88	1·33	1·42	2·48
Expected	11·17	7·45	17·38	

*in thousands

The incidence rate of tendinitis cases for the entire plant can be easily computed using the OSHA formula:

$$\text{Incidence rate} = \frac{\text{Cases} \times 200{,}000}{\text{Hours worked}}$$

---

[c]Material supplied by M. Keyserling, same plant Z data as presented in Chapter 5.

By substituting data from Table C5, the rate for the entire plant was found to be 2·48. The incidence rates of tendinitis in each department were also computed and are presented in the table.

A cursory analysis shows that the rate of tendinitis cases in Department A was more than three times that in Departments B or C. The statistical test, discussed below, can be used to compare rates among the departments.

Statistical method for identifying problem areas

To determine whether differences exist in the incidence rates of tendinitis in the three departments at Plant Z, it is necessary to test the null hypothesis,

where:

$$H_o: \quad I_A = I_B = I_C$$

I_A = incidence rate in Department A,
I_B = incidence rate in Department B,
I_C = incidence rate in Department C,

against the alternative hypothesis,

where:

$$H_1: \quad \text{Not all } I_i \text{ are equal.}$$

Duncan described a nonparametric approach for testing the null hypothesis.[8] The method computes a Chi-square statistic according to the following formula:

$$\chi^2_{m-1} = \sum_{i=1}^{m} \frac{(E_i - O_i)^2}{E_i}$$

χ^2 = test statistic with $(m-1)$ degrees of freedom,
m = number of groups being compared (in this case, $m = 3$),
E_i = expected number of incidents in group i,
O_i = observed number of incidents in group i,
$i = 1, 2, 3, \ldots m$.

The value of E_i is computed using the following equation where:

$$E_i = \frac{H_i \times O_T}{H_T}$$

H_i = hours of exposure in group i,
H_T = total hours of exposure for all groups,
O_T = total observed incidents for all groups.

A restriction on this test is that the expected number of incidents in each group (E_i) must be at least five.[9]

Substituting the appropriate entries from Table C5 into the above equations, the Chi-square test statistic was computed to be 15·1, which is significant at the 0·01 level. This means that it is highly improbable that the recorded incident rates for the three departments are equivalent. Since they are not equivalent, there must be some factor(s) that is (are) responsible for the higher incident rates occurring in Department A that may not be occurring in Departments B and C. Based on the expected values shown Table C5, and the computed incidence rate for each of the three departments, the conclusion is that Department A should be further investigated to determine the causes of the larger incidence of tendinitis.

The Chi-square test described above was appropriate in this example because the total number of tendinitis cases in Plant Z (36) and the distribution of exposure hours in the three departments resulted in values of E_i that exceeded 5. Unfortunately, this requirement is not met in many settings because population sizes are smaller. In situations like these, it is often necessary to make decisions without conclusive results of statistical tests.

Postscript

International Perspective: some CTD prevention strategies

Although in the United States the label "cumulative trauma disorder" is the most common term used to refer to these problems, it is evident from the scientific literature that problems similar to CTDs, whether referred to as repetitive strain injuries, occupational cervico-brachial disorders, or occupational overuse syndromes, are growing problems in every major industrialized country*. This is most evident from reports carried in the media and medical literature. With the exception of Sweden, Australia, and perhaps the United States, it is unclear if other countries with high-risk work populations have implemented any special guidelines for these disorders, or amended existing occupational health and safety regulations to cover the work-related musculoskeletal disorders. The three countries that have taken a more direct approach to the problem each illustrate a type of prevention strategy that was designed to fit the prevention needs of the individual country.

Sweden in 1984 issued a regulation titled: "Ordinance concerning work postures and working environment."[10] This ordinance, prepared by the National Board of Occupational Safety and Health in Sweden, represents the first attempt by any country to provide legislation for controlling CTDs. The ordinance consists of 7 Sections, each specifying one or more provisions concerning work postures, working environment and physical load. Rather than account for every work contingency, the provisions were developed to indicate general principles for the implementation of the Work Environment Act in Sweden. The following excerpt from Section 1 illustrates the nature and spirit of the ordinance:

> Work must be designed so as to avoid unnecessarily fatiguing or otherwise strenuous work postures and working movements. Efforts must be made to enable the person doing the work to vary his work posture and working movements. If there is little opportunity of variation, the person doing the work must be given suitably disposed breaks.

---

*Because of the confusion in both terminology and diagnostic categories in identifying work-related musculoskeletal disorders, a select group of participants from the international health community (World Health Organization) plan to meet in 1988 to consider some common terminology and diagnostic criteria for labelling these conditions.

Although the ordinance does not contain an ergonomic equivalent of a "threshold limit value", or similar quantitative values for controlling biomechanical stress at the workplace, it does provide a set of useful recommendations and explanations for good ergonomic work practices.

Australia, in a similar fashion, developed a "Model Code of Practice" in response to what was seen as a near epidemic of musculoskeletal problems among a number of high risk occupations in their country that included packers, sorters, machinists and keyboard operators.[11] In early 1980 a tripartite special Commission was formed to draft a report on ways to prevent repetitive motion injury (RSI), the Australian equivalent of the cumulative trauma disorders. The report was released in 1986, published for the National Occupational Health and Safety Commission, "Worksafe Australia", by Australian Government Publishing Service.

The objective of the Australian Model Code of Practice was to provide a framework for minimizing the risk of, and management of, RSI. The proposed prevention strategy consists of recommendations covering eight main elements or factors including the following: work organization, job and task design, task variation/work pauses, work adjustment periods, workplace and environment design, technology selection, equipment design and education and training.

The philosophy and content of the Australian Code of Practice parallels the Swedish ordinance. For example, Item 1 of the Australian Code stresses the need for work "to be organized so that employees are able to regulate some of the pressures related to their work." Likewise, the Swedish ordinance suggests that "efforts must be made to arrange work in such a way that the employee can influence his own working structure" (Work Environment Act, Ch. 2, Section 1, Subsection 2).

In the **United States**, the National Institute for Occupational Safety and Health (NIOSH) in cooperation with the Association of Schools of Public Health, completed a Proposed National Strategy for Preventing Musculoskeletal Injuries in 1985.[12,13] Unlike the Australian and Swedish documents, the U.S. National Strategy focussed more on the process for preventing musculoskeletal disorders than on specific recommendations. The musculoskeletal strategy identified research and informational needs, such as: (1) the need for better surveillance and diagnostic information for identifying the disorders, (2) the types of research that needed to be done, and (3) the role of the public and private sectors in implementing and evaluating the proposed interventions. Of the different interventions considered, a main conclusion was that ergonomic changes in the form of job and tool redesign should be attempted first, and that training and employee selection should be secondary. The strategy also stressed the importance of dissemination to ensure that needed target groups receive the information on the implementation of successful interventions for reducing CTDs. Implementation would be facilitated by the establishment of a National Committee and Clearinghouse that would promote interchange of information.

Other than the guidelines found in this Manual, there are no other recommended, official or unofficial, work practices or codes in the U.S. for controlling CTDs in the workplace. In the related area of lifting, NIOSH-sponsored and published a *Work Practices Guide for Manual Lifting* in 1981, which is to be updated and expanded in 1988 to include a wider variety of lifting conditions.[14] The revised lifting guide, like its predecessors, provides only recommendations or guidelines that are neither standards nor designed to be used for enforcement of safe work behavior. This approach appears to reflect a general philosophy that compliance will occur voluntarily when both management and workers recognize that it is in their best interest, from both a health and economic stand point, to cooperate in reducing work-related injury and lost time. One way to facilitate this process is to provide the necessary information about these disorders and their prevention, which is a goal of this manual.

References—Appendices

1. Cyriax, J., 1982, Diagnosis of Soft Tissue Lesions, *Textbook of Orthopaedic Medicine*. (Philadelphia, PA: Bailliere-Tindall (Saunders)), 8th ed., Vol 1, 1–61.
2. MacMachon, B. and Pugh, T.F., 1970, *Epidemiology: Principles and Methods*, (Boston: Little, Brown and Company).
3. U.S. Department of Labor, Annual Survey of Occupational Injuries and Illnesses, 1981, In: *Handbook of Methods*, Bureau of Labor Statistics, Bulletin 2134–1, Chapter 17. Occupational Safety and Health Statistics, 122–134.
4. American National Standards Institute, 1969, *Methods for Recording and Measuring Work Injury Experience*, Standard No. Z16.1, (New York: American National Standard).
5. Jensen, R.C., Klein, B.P. and Sanderson, L.M., 1983, Motion-related wrist disorders traced to industries, occupational groups. *Monthly Labor Review*, (Sept.) 13–16.
6. Armstrong, T., Foulke, J., Joseph, B. and Goldstein, S., 1982, Investigation of cumulative trauma disorders in a poultry processing plant. *Am. Ind. Hyg. Assoc. J.*, **43,** 103–116.
7. Keyserling, W.M., Donoghue, J., Punnett, L., and Miller, A., 1982, *Repetitive Trauma Disorders in the Garment Industry*. (National Institute for Occupational Safety and Health: Final Report).
8. Duncan, D., 1955, Multiply range and multiple F tests. *Biometrics,* **11,** 1–42.
9. Fleiss, J., 1981, *Statistical Methods for Rates and Proportions*. 2nd edition, (New York: John Wiley).
10. Danielson, G., Edstrom, R. and Lindh, G., 1984, Ordinance concerning Work Postures and Working Movements, *National Board of Occupational Safety and Health*. Stockholm, Sweden.
11. National Occupational Health and Safety Commission, 1986, "Repetitive Strain Injury (RSI): A Report and Model Code of Practice." *Worksafe Australia*, (Canberra: Australian Government Publishing Service).
12. Proposed National Strategies for the Prevention of Leading Work-Related Diseases and Injuries, Part 1, 1986 (Washington, D.C.: the Association of Schools of Public Health under a cooperative agreement with the National Institute for Occupational Safety and Health). (NTIS (ID No. 87 114 740).
13. Millar, J.D., 1988 Summary of Proposed National Strategies for the Prevention of Leading Work-Related Diseases and Injuries. *American Journal of Industrial Medicine*, **13,** 223–240.
14. *Work Practices Guide for Manual Lifting*, 1981, NIOSH Technical Report, (Cincinnati, OH: DHHS Publication No. 81–122).

Suggested Reading

Psychology of Change

Dalton, M., 1950, Conflicts between staff and line managerial officers. *American Sociological Review.* **15,** 342–351.

Hopkins, B.L. and Sears, J., 1982, Managing behavior for productivity. In *Handbook of Organizational Behavior Management.* Edited by L.W. Fredericksen (New York: John Wiley).

Kotter, J.P. and Schlesinger, L.A., 1979, Choosing strategies for change. *Harvard Business Review.* March April, pp. 106–113.

Kanter, R.M., 1983, *The Change Masters.* (New York: Simon and Schuster).

Koch, L. and French, J.R., 1948, Overcoming resistance to change. *Human Relations* **1,** 512–532.

Smith, L.A. and Smith J.L., 1982, How can an IE justify a human factors activities program to management? *Industrial Engineering.* **14**(2), 39–43.

Ergonomics: General

Note: Portions of this ergonomics bibliography were made available by The Human Factors Society, P.O. Box 1369, Santa Monica, CA 90406. Our thanks to them for providing this information.

Armstrong, T. and Kochhar, D., 1982, Work performance and handicapped persons. In: *Industrial Engineering Handbook* edited by G. Salvendy. (New York: John Wiley).

Eastman Kodak Company, Human Factors Section, 1983, *Ergonomic Design For People at Work* (Belmont, CA: Lifetime Learning Publications) Vol. 1.

Eastman Kodak Company, Ergonomics Group., 1986, *Ergonomic Design For People at Work.* (New York: Van Nostrand Reinhold Co.) Vol. 2.

Chaffin, D.B. and Andersson, G.B.J., 1984, *Occupational Biomechanics.* (New York: John Wiley).

Grandjean, E., 1980, *Fitting the task to the Man: An Ergonomic Approach.* (London: Taylor & Francis Ltd.) (3rd. ed).

Hertzberg, H.T., 1960, Dynamic anthropometry or working positions. *Human Factors,* **2**(3), 147–155.

Huchingson, R.D., 1981, *New Horizons for Human Factors Design.* (New York: McGraw Hill).

McCormick, E.J. and Sanders, M.S., 1982, *Human Factors in Engineering and Design* (New York: McGraw Hill) (5th ed).

Murell, K.F.H., 1980, *Ergonomics: Man in His Working Environment.* (London: Chapman & Hall).

Oborne, D.J., 1982, *Ergonomics At Work.* (New York: John Wiley).

Shackel, B., 1974, (Editor), *Applied Ergonomics Handbook.* (Guildford: IPC Science and Technology Press).

Singleton, W.T., 1972, *Introduction to Ergonomics.* (Geneva: World

Health Organization). Distributed by Q Corporation, 49 Sheridan Ave., Albany, NY 12210.

Tichauer, E.R., 1978, *The Biomechanical Basis of Ergonomics*. (New York: John Wiley).

U.S. Department of Defense, 1981, *Human Engineering Design Criteria for Military Systems, Equipment, and Facilities* (MIL-STD-1472C). Available from Naval Publications and Forms Center, 5801 Tabor Ave., Philadelphia, PA 19120.

Woodson, W.E., 1981, *Human Factors Design Handbook*. (New York: McGraw-Hill).

Worker characteristics

Chaffin, D.B., 1975, Ergonomics Guide For the Assessment of Human Static Strength. *American Industrial Hygiene Association Journal.* **36,** 505–511.

Diffrient, N., Tilley, A.R., Harman, D. and Bardagjy, J.C., 1981, *Humanscale*. (Cambridge, MA: MIT Press). (A useful collection of human dimensions for design.)

Hunt, V.R., 1979, *Work and the Health of Women*. (Boca Raton, FL: CRC Press.)

Laubach, L.L., 1976, Comparative Muscular Strength of Men and Women: A Review of the Literature. *Aviation, Space, and Environmental Medicine* **47**(5), 534–542.

National Aeronautics and Space Administration, 1978, *Anthropometric Source Book* (NASA Reference Publication 1024). (Washington, D.C.: NASA) (Vols. I, II, III).

Singleton, W.T., 1983, (Editor) *The Body at Work*. (Cambridge: Cambridge University Press).

Sleight, R.B. and Cook, K.G., 1974, *Problems in Occupational Safety and Health: A Critical Review of Select Worker Physical and Psychological Factors* (HEW Publication No. [NIOSH] 75–124). (Washington, D.C.: U.S. Government Printing Office).

Welford, A.T., 1976, Thirty Years of Psychological Research on Age and Work. *Journal of Occupational Psychology.* **49,** 129–138.

Job design

AIHA Technical Committee on Ergonomics, 1970, Ergonomics Guide to Assessment of Metabolic and Cardiac Costs of Physical Work. *American Industrial Hygiene Association Journal.* **32,** 560–564.

Helander, M., 1981, *Human Factors/Ergonomics For Building and Construction*. (New York: John Wiley).

Konz, S., 1979, *Work Design*. (Columbus, OH: Grid Pub. Inc.).

Salvendy, G. and Smith, M.J., 1981, *Machine Pacing and Occupational Stress*. (London: Taylor & Francis Ltd.).

U.S. Department of Health and Human Services, 1981, *Work Practices Guide for Manual Lifting* (DHSS [NIOSH] Publication No. 81–122). (Cincinnati, OH: NIOSH) (March).

Equipment design

Alden, D.G., Daniels, R.W. and Kanarick, A.F., 1972, Keyboard Design and Operation: A Review of the Major Issues. *Human Factors* **14**(4), 275–293.

Armstrong, T.J., 1983, *An Ergonomics Guide to Carpal Tunnel Syndrome*. (Akron, OH: American Industrial Hygiene Association).

Damon, A., Stoudt, H.W. and McFarland, R.A., 1966, *The Human Body in Equipment Design*. (Cambridge, MA: Harvard University Press).

Fraser, T.M., 1980, *Ergonomic Principles in the Design of Hand Tools.* (Occupational Safety and Health Series No. 44). (Geneva, Switzerland: International Labor Office).

Greenberg, L. and Chaffin, D.B., 1977, *Workers and Their Tools.* (Midland, MI: Pendell).

Kroemer, K.H.E., 1983, *Ergonomics of VDT Workplaces.* (Akron, OH: American Industrial Hygiene Association).

Sauter, S.L., Chapman, L.J. and Knutson, S.J., 1984, *Improving VDT Work: Causes and Control of Health Concerns in VDT Use.* (Lawrence, Kansas: The Report Store).

Tichauer, E.R. and Gage, H., 1977, Ergonomic Principles Basic to Hand Tool Design. *American Industrial Hygiene Association Journal.* **38,** 622–634.

Van Cott, H.P. and Kinkade, R.G., 1972, (editors) *Human Engineering Guide to Equipment Design* (Washington, D.C: U.S. Government Printing Office) (revised edition).

Workplace design

Ayoub, M.M., 1973, Work place Design and Posture. *Human Factors,* **15**(3), 265–268.

Chaffin, D.B., 1973, Localized Muscle Fatigue—Definition and Measurement. *Journal of Occupational Medicine.* **15**(4), 346–354.

Kroemer, K.H.E., 1971, Seating in Plant and Office. *American Industrial Hygiene Association Journal.* **32,** 633–652.

Kvalseth, T.O., 1983, *Ergonomics of Workstation Design.* (London: Butterworths).

Roebuck, Jr., J.A., Kroemer, K.H.E. and Thomson, W.G., 1975, *Engineering Anthropometry Methods.* (New York: John Wiley).

Environmental design

Illuminating Engineering Society, 1979, *American National Standard Practice for Industrial Lighting* (ANSI Standard RP–7–1979). (New York: Illuminating Engineering Society).

National Institute for Occupational Safety and Health, 1984, Vibration Syndrome in Chipping and Grinding Workers. *J. Occ. Med.,* **26**(10), 765–788.

Parker, J.F. and West, V.R., 1973, *Bioastronautics Data Book* (NASA SP–3006) (Washington, D.C: U.S. Government Printing Office). (2nd edition).

Poulton, E.C., 1972, *Environment and Human Efficiency.* (Springfield, IL: Charles C. Thomas).

U.S. Department of Health, Education, and Welfare, 1973, *The Industrial Environment—Its Evaluation and Control.* (Washington, D.C: U.S. Government Printing Office (NIOSH).